Old School Medicine

Lower tech care to improve
the ***high tech*** future
of ***healthcare***

Linda R. Thompson, M.D.

Old School Medicine
Lower tech care to improve the high tech future of healthcare
by Linda R. Thompson, M.D.

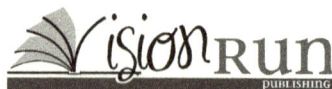

VISIONRUN PUBLISHING

305 PORTSMOUTH RD
KNOXVILLE TN 37909
VISIONRUN.COM

Linda R. Thompson, MD

*This book is dedicated to the
Class of 1966 at the
University of Virginia Medical School
and all of our teachers at the time we
were there*

Old School Medicine

CONTENTS

Old School Medicine

CHAPTER ONE

Introduction

"Time," said the famous Athenian general Pericles, "is the wisest counselor of all." And so it is with the perspective of time that I review — through the pages that follow — the changes, innovations and even a few disasters that have emerged in the practice of medicine, particularly in the area of mental health. I have been working as a psychiatrist full time since graduating from medical school in 1966, completing a rotating internship in 1967, and completing my residency in June of 1971. Most of my work has been in private practice, although I have also done quite a bit of consulting with mental health centers during that time as well.

Coincidentally, the year I began practicing ('71) could also be called the beginning of the digital age. The first microprocessor was invented, as was email. At that time, these inventions were minor stories in the scientific community that grew like a mushroom cloud over the next several decades, impacting almost every area of our lives, especially in the sciences. Over the span of my career, those advances in technology changed the face of medicine. But as you likely know, not all change is good. Some changes have unintended consequences, and I'll be highlighting and discussing those.

But we in the medical community have also changed the way we teach and train physicians aside from the technological advances. I'll be addressing the implications of those changes as well. Today there are significant problems in the delivery of treatments to patients, and some very effective treatment strategies have been abandoned in the process of change. From this insider's viewpoint, there are multiple reasons why the American healthcare system is the most expensive in the world and why the results of the current delivery of services provides more limited outcomes in spite of all those dollars. There is also more we can and should consider, especially ways to simplify and humanize the system, which is the reason for this book.

A word about privacy and patient confidentiality — I will be providing many clinical examples throughout the book. They are all true stories, but in the interest of privacy I have combined some patients into a single clinical example to disguise individual identities. None of these examples should be seen as identifying an actual person, living or dead. In describing patients' histories and outcomes, I'll be choosing first names that are the only fictional part of the example.

Each of the stories presented taught me something important in the course of my development as a physician. They are not necessarily a chronological account of my actual studies during medical school, internship and residency, just the ones that were important to my growth.

During my second year of college, I decided to become a physician. Even though I had enrolled as a pre-med major, it was only because that would allow me to transfer to any other major after two years without losing any time toward graduation. There were two other students in my class who intended to go to medical school, and I gradually decided to continue in pre-med and apply to medical school after graduation. The economy at the time was still somewhat unstable and we were in the early stages of the Vietnam War. I felt there would always be a need for good doctors no matter what was happening to the economy. It was a decision born of pragmatism as much as calling.

Pearl Harbor was attacked when I was just 6 months old, and I grew up in the aftermath of World War II. My father told me many times that he had been shaving when he got the call about Pearl Harbor. He was a newspaper reporter. On hearing the news, he immediately wiped the shaving cream off the unshaven half of his face and rushed into the office with his face half shaven. That's how important the story was, to him as a reporter, as well as to the country. My mother's only brother died in a submarine in the South Pacific sometime in early 1943. I have five younger siblings and as a family we struggled somewhat financially. However we never went without the basic necessities and we learned responsibility early, for which I am grateful. As I grew up, my parents told us stories about the hard times they had during the Great Depression, and I was very aware that having a stable profession would always be important to having a stable income.

I considered the possibility of graduate school during my first two years of college, and decided it was not for me. The idea of writing a masters' thesis and possibly a doctoral dissertation did not appeal to me. Besides, I reasoned, if we were to plunge into another deep economic depression, I was not sure that a graduate degree without specialized skills would be all that helpful, so it seemed impractical.

CHAPTER TWO

Medical School: The Pre-Clinical Years

Once I was in medical school, I was sure I'd made the right choice of profession, and clinical rotations in the third and fourth years further confirmed to me that I had made the right decision. My undergraduate studies paved the way for entrance into the University of Virginia's medical school, an excellent program. The evaluation and treatment of patients was fascinating and endlessly challenging work. For the most part I had excellent teachers but I also learned an enormous amount from the patients themselves and from their families as well.

I don't remember exactly when I learned that there were two different types of students in medical school. It was probably in an informal discussion during or after morning rounds or late afternoon staffing when those on call were getting caught up on the new admissions and problems with current patients. There were book learners who took care of their patients during the day, went to Grand Rounds and lectures and then spent the rest of their day in the library or their rooms reading about the illnesses and treatments they were learning about.

Grand Rounds were another learning opportunity. These were hospital-wide assemblies of physicians, nurses and other medical staff, at all levels of training and expertise, and they generally take place in a large auditorium or assemble hall. These are generally done on a weekly basis, and a specific patient's illness and/or treatment would be presented to those in attendance.

And there were case learners, who also attended Grand Rounds and lectures and then spent most of the rest of their time hanging out on the wards and learning medicine in a more hands-on approach. They also studied, but most of their learning occurred in the context of individual patients and their illnesses and treatments. There were always appropriate texts on the units that you could refer to quickly if there was a particular issue to sort through. This was the trade school approach and it was a perfect fit for me.

When I was in medical school, the patient would sometimes be present for the Grand Rounds presentation, if that was appropriate, and if the patient was stable enough to attend the meeting. This was another important part of the education of students and house staff and allowed more senior clinicians to provide information about the newest challenges or latest treatments for a given malady. This was also helpful in the ongoing learning of generalist and specialist doctors who were no longer in formal training.

The most important course prior to starting into the clinical years was the course in how to take a comprehensive history and perform a thorough physical examination. All the other courses of the first two years were devoted to the basic sciences that provided the scientific basis for the practice of medicine. But the history and physical examination were the primary tools for the initial assessment of the patient's illness and they were to lead to the decisions about which tests and procedures were needed to rule in or out the initial diagnosis that was being considered for the individual patient. Following the write-up of the history and physical, we were to write a formulation of the patient's presentation, including all relevant data and information, thus summarizing the important elements of the history and physical that led to the specific diagnosis or diagnoses of the patient's illness. This usually took an additional 1/3 to one page of the initial write-up of the patient's presentation and illness, and this would have to be defended to the residents and attending physicians on rounds later that day or on morning rounds on the following day. Recommendations for lab tests, x-rays, diagnostic procedures and the initial treatment would end the write-up, and would also have to be defended in rounds. We were expected to be able to list the most likely diagnoses for each patient and to be able to accurately diagnose the more common ailments. We could put down a list of rule/out diagnoses in situations where the diagnosis was less certain. It was expected that we would usually have a good sense of the patient's diagnosis and treatment by the end of taking the history and physical examination. And in cases where the diagnosis was not clear, we were to at least have reasonable ideas for obtaining an accurate diagnosis out of the range of possibilities elicited by the history and physical examination.

A majority of the cases were fairly routine and did not require a lot of discussion. However, there was a significant minority of patients whose presentations were not as clear, and a lot could be learned by the questions and input of the more experienced house staff and attending physicians. Our daily clinical notes described additions to our thinking on the patient, and the results of discussions coming out of the daily rounds. These, together with the additional information available from labs and procedures, gave us an ongoing history of the patient's changing status as well as their response to treatment. Final notes would be done at the time of discharge or death and would provide a summary of the patient's initial presentation, hospital course, response to treatment and status at the end of the hospitalization.

This course was taught in the second semester of the second year, which for me was in the spring of 1964. Naturally we did not have the multitude of sophisticated tests and procedures that we have available now. Some of the treatments we had then were relatively new, such as the anti-anxiety and anti-depressant medications in psychiatry. Antibiotics had been around for roughly 20+ years and had changed the outcomes for many infectious diseases. Anti-cancer drugs were coming into routine use, but the field of oncology or cancer treatment was still in its early stages. Surgical treatments for cancer were what we used to call "commando procedures," which basically meant taking out most of the tissue surrounding the cancer in the hopes of "getting it all." Compared to today's surgeries, these were frequently mutilating and involved taking out everything in the area that was not necessary for living. Radiation treatments were also coming into routine use. Side effects were very difficult with both treatment types, and the unfolding of their development over the past 50 years has been in the direction of more focused treatments for many cancers, with less aggressive surgical interventions as well.

Patients were usually hospitalized for significantly longer than they are now and treatments could be initiated and followed for several weeks before they were transitioned to outpatient care. Surgical patients were typically hospitalized for 7 to 10 days with appendectomies or gall bladder surgeries. Cancer patients could be hospitalized for several months when they had extensive surgeries, and when the surgery was to be followed by chemotherapy and/or radiation.

Psychiatric patients were routinely hospitalized for three to four months and six to twelve months was not unusual, especially if they didn't get a good response to the initial medication trials. In that case, changes would be required in an effort to achieve a better outcome. When a patient's treatment was insured, the insurance would typically cover three to four months of inpatient treatment. If the insurance coverage ran out before the patient was recovered enough for discharge, they would be transferred to the state hospital for an indefinite period of time for additional treatment. In rare instances, a patient would be transferred back to our unit for more active treatment prior to final discharge. With the increasing changes in insurance reimbursements and the push to have patients discharged at the earliest possible time, the various fields of medicine, including psychiatry, have undergone a transition to less comprehensive histories and physicals, and an insistence (by the insurance companies) on a single primary diagnosis, for which providers are paid a set fee. There is little support for more complicated cases, or for patients receiving the comprehensive and trial based treatments that were routine during my medical training. And while the insurance companies are trying to contain costs of treatment at every turn, the design of the modern hospital has led to more expensive, all private rooms for patients, and we have discarded the more efficient and therapeutic open wards that were the standard of care in most hospitals in the country until the 1960s and early 1970s. Patients may be more comfortable during their brief stays, but they are not better served because of the upgrades. In fact, just the opposite is true. They are more isolated in the private rooms and chronic understaffing of medical units leaves them with long delays of getting help from nursing staff when needed as well as less time generally with medical caregivers.

CHAPTER THREE

Medical School – The Clinical Years

My first clinical rotation was in pediatrics. As part of that rotation we went by bus to Lynchburg, Virginia where the Lynchburg Colony was located. This was where infants were sent who had severe intellectual and/or physical disabilities. Many of them were placed there as newborns when something significantly disabling was identified. The parents had the choice of whether to place the baby in state care for the rest of their lives or try to take care of them as best they could at home. Most of the children had Down's syndrome with severe mental retardation. We spent most of our time in the infants' and children's wards. However we also saw adult wards of the state, who had resided there all their lives, walking in groups out on the grounds of the facility. The staff appeared to provide excellent care for all the wards.

When we were in the toddlers' playroom we saw very active children playing under staff supervision and most of them were interested in us. They did not communicate verbally, but would come close to look at us quickly before going back to playing as before.

One of the staff led us into the room where the children slept, because there was a child there she wanted us to see. He was a thalidomide baby, placed in state custody as a newborn. Thalidomide was a drug manufactured in Germany that was in use for insomnia and anxiety. It was mostly used as a sedative. It had not yet been released for general use in the US. However, there were samples of the medication being used on a trial basis in the US. This child's mother was apparently given samples of thalidomide to take during her pregnancy. Her child was born with fingers coming out of one of his shoulders and only part of the other arm and hand. His legs were also deformed, but not as severely as his arms. The mortality of infants born after this exposure during the pregnancy was 40 - 50%. There were other severe abnormalities in many of these children, including heart defects. The staff member wanted us to see this particular child because for all of his disabilities, she did not think he was retarded.

When we gathered around his crib, he began to cry because he recognized us as strangers and was afraid of us. He was about 18 months old and spent most of his time in his crib, because he was not independently mobile. The chairman of pediatrics was with us on this trip and he assessed the boy and realized that he was, indeed, not mentally challenged. He spent some time talking to all of us about the significance of stranger anxiety, which is normal in most infants between eight to fourteen months of age, and episodically after that if there is significant disruption in the primary parental bond during this period. Children who are severely retarded do not form the normal exclusive bond with a parent, usually the mother, because of their developmental limitations. This boy had clearly bonded with one or more of his regular caretakers, and he was frightened by us because he knew we were strangers. The chairman arranged for the child to be transferred to the Children's Rehabilitation Center, which was just outside Charlottesville and a part of the University.

While I did not know it at the time, I have since realized that this move was a significant loss for him, because while it was medically appropriate, it separated him from his initial caretakers. During my third year of residency, he was still at the rehab center when I was there for a brief visit with the Child and Adolescent service. He was undergoing multiple surgeries to allow him to be as independent as possible. I saw him at a distance, working with a woman on the staff who was assisting him. He was in a wheelchair with braces on his legs, and appeared to be in good spirits and very comfortable in the setting of the rehab center. I was glad to see that he seemed to have adjusted well. By that time, he was about six or seven years old.

Thalidomide was never authorized for use in the US. However, it continues to be used in Europe. The children who were born with these terrible birth defects were a small minority of the infants exposed to thalidomide during their fetal development. It was later determined that the mothers of the affected infants had taken thalidomide at a time when they were deficient in one or more of the B vitamins, and it was this combination that led to the terrible deformities.

My third year of medical school training included two-month rotations on medicine, pediatrics, psychiatry and general surgery. By the end of the year I knew I was going into psychiatry. There were changes taking place in both medicine and the format for medical education. For the first time, it became possible to create electives during the fourth year, and these electives could be taken at the University hospital or at another medical school if we chose. Quite a few of my classmates took advantage of this to get electives in areas they were interested in specializing in. I did not choose to take these electives, and stayed with the regular courses for my fourth year. My reasoning for this decision was that I knew I had only seen the tip of the iceberg that represented all of medicine and I felt it was way too soon to move into more specialized medicine. Again, I think this was partly a result of my being a case learner, and I wanted to be sure I was a good physician generally before I entered my residency years. I did do an externship in psychiatry during the summer between my third and fourth years, and continued to learn more about that field without missing any of the fourth year courses.

During my fourth year, most of my rotations were one month in length and contained several surgical subspecialties in addition to a month of neurology and additional regular medicine and surgical rotations. The most important case I saw during that year was a young man who was sent to us from a rural county in Virginia, because he needed to have his aortic valve replaced on an emergency basis. He had been healthy until about a month before he was admitted. This happened over a weekend and I was on call that weekend. I watched while the senior and first year cardiovascular residents worked him up rapidly and then called the chairman of the department to report on his condition. He was in his late twenties and when I first saw him I was astounded by his color. He was severely cyanotic, which means his skin was a dark, bluish-purple. That bluish coloring indicates a lack of adequate oxygen, as well as high carbon dioxide levels, yet he was on maximum oxygen. As it turned out, instead of a tricuspid aortic valve, he had a bicuspid aortic valve, (an inherited form of heart disease) which was essentially destroyed at that point by an infection, known as acute bacterial endocarditis.

The heart normally has a tricuspid valve, one with three leaflets, which will close tightly after the heart's left ventricle pumps the oxygenated blood out of the heart and into the main artery, the aorta. When the heart relaxes to allow the newly oxygenated blood to enter the ventricle from the left atrium, the aortic valve closes tightly so no blood leaks back into the heart from the aorta. Bicuspid valves are reasonably common and can be relatively benign, but they are more vulnerable to becoming infected if there is a bacterial spread through the vascular system. This can occur after dental procedures and even minor surgical procedures if the individual is not pre-medicated prior to the procedures. The patient didn't know about the problem with his heart valve until he became ill with the endocarditis.

When I first saw him, he was sitting on the edge of his bed, with his feet propped up on the bed frame, and his arms were wrapped around his knees, holding them as close to his chest as possible. He was taking rapid breaths as hard as he could and he could never get enough oxygen into his body, because almost all of the blood his heart would pump out to the aorta, would fall back into the ventricle when the heart muscle relaxed. He was sweating profusely from the exertion of breathing so hard and his hospital gown and the bed sheets around him were soaked through. He couldn't talk because all of his effort had to go into breathing as fast as he could. He could nod or shake his head to yes/no questions, which was the only way he could communicate. He was rapidly prepped for surgery and the chairman came in to do the valve replacement. I will never forget the desperation in that man's eyes as he was slowly suffocating before our eyes. The resident told me after the surgery that he was no more than one to two hours from death at the time he arrived. It was late fall in 1965, and heart surgery was a very new field. It was not usually available outside of a university medical center. If the patient had developed the same infection two or three years earlier, he would have died from it, in the agonizing state that he was in at admission. Fortunately for him, he received a new heart valve that day, survived the surgery and was able to return home in good health.

He was in the ICU for several days before he was stable enough to be transferred to one of the regular floors. During that time, he started having hallucinations, and the staff was concerned about this. It is now known that it's not uncommon for patients in the ICU to become transiently psychotic, which is frequently part of a delirium, but can occur for other reasons as well. Also by this time, it was generally known that I was going into psychiatry when I finished my internship. So they asked me to see him and let them know what I thought.

After introducing myself as a medical student, I asked him if he had been seeing things that weren't real and he said that he was. When I asked him to describe them, he said he saw them on the ceiling, sort of like movies. He said they didn't scare him. He denied hearing any voices or other sounds that didn't seem real. As I was thinking for a moment about what to ask next, he got this grin on his face. He looked me in the eye and said, "I know that you all think I'm crazy for seeing these things. But I'm stuck here in this bed. I can't get up yet. And they kind of entertain me while I have to lay here. I know they're not real. But I don't worry about that. Because now I can breathe, really breathe, and that is all I care about. I'm really OK with this." I had to smile. Yes, I told him, I thought he was OK too, and wished him well for when he returned home. Within a few days, I would be going off the service and since he was not one of my assigned patients, I wouldn't be seeing him again. But I have never forgotten him. To this day, he has defined severe air hunger for me.

I have only seen one other patient with that dark cyanosis and that was in an elderly man with severe terminal lung disease. However, I recently read John Barry's book, *The Great Influenza*, and there are descriptions of this kind of dark cyanosis in many of the victims, especially the healthy young adults that died during the 1918 influenza. He reports these cases as usually dying from the effects of the body's attempts to kill off the infection in the lungs, creating severe damage to lung tissue and an inability to get enough oxygen into the body to sustain life. It is a fascinating account of a severe pandemic and well worth reading.

The other important rotation for me was the rotation on chest surgery. In one of the lectures during my first two years of medical school, the lecturer gave us the following statistics: Out of each graduating class from medical school, one member would be lost to suicide, one to alcohol and/or drug abuse and one to tuberculosis. My class started with 77 students. At that point in history, we had all grown up experiencing polio epidemics, and most of us knew people who either had the disease, or had died from it. Tuberculosis was mostly contained in sanitariums, so we were less familiar with it; but exposure to infectious diseases was seen by most of us as just a hazard of the profession, and of life in general. So while the statistics quoted may seem startling to today's reader, they were not terribly surprising to us at the time.

In fact there was a story that made the rounds when I was in med school (and I have no way of knowing whether it was truth or exaggeration, but it is certainly plausible) about a doctor doing an autopsy on a cadaver that was believed to have died of pneumonia. But on inspection, the patient had died of the Bubonic Plague, which is 100% fatal in the pneumonia form. Exposure to the deadly disease, even from the cadaver, took the life of the examining doctor as well. Today people freak out because there are antibiotic-resistant bugs out there. But that was part of the deal back then.

At times now we appear to have forgotten that death is not a problem to be solved. It's something that will happen to all of us at some point and we just need to learn how to deal with it.

The way we have nearly conquered the infectious disease piece changed medicine in so many ways. Many of the things we as doctors would ordinarily have been exposed to have been taken out of the mix. We've become a bit arrogant as a result.

While I was on chest surgery I scrubbed in on procedures to collapse the chest wall over the part of the lung that continued to be infected with the mycobacterium tuberculosis. The procedure sounds primitive by today's medical standards. It involved breaking a couple of ribs below the collarbone and collapsing the chest wall over the top of one or both lungs, where the infection resided. It was done in order to take the burden of breathing off that diseased part of the lung, and allow it to have a chance to heal. It caused a deformity, but people were willing to go through it not to have to die in the hospital. Back then, everyone with active tuberculosis was required by law to remain in a sanitarium until they had three consecutive sputum cultures that were negative for the bacterium. Only then could they return home to their families.

After the surgery, we would do rounds on these patients and would have to suction them to pull out any mucus that might lead to a secondary infection of pneumonia. This would also make them cough very intensely and they would bring up more sputum. The surgery was mutilating, and experimental. But some of these patients had been in the sanitarium for several years, and they desperately wanted to be out in the world again. They did not want to die in the sanitarium. As I talked to some of them about their experiences in the sanitarium, I found the stories to be very sad for the most part.

All of us had to have TB tests regularly. One of our lecturers in medical school said that 10% of the average class would have a positive tuberculin test at the time they started medical school, and they would be followed by X-rays to check for infection with tuberculosis. Eighty per cent of the class would convert to a positive TB test during medical school and they would be followed by X-rays and sputum cultures as well. If they had a positive sputum test, they would have to go to the sanitarium for treatment. Fortunately, by the time I finished medical school, there were effective drugs to treat and cure tuberculosis so that if you developed a positive TB test, you would be started on one of these drugs for a year and would be checked for disease by X-rays only. In spite of my exposure during that month, I remained among the 10% of the class that did not convert to a positive TB test.

The other significant event of my fourth year was my decision to take a rotating internship after graduation and then return to the University of Virginia for my psychiatric residency. Rotating internships were falling out of favor at that time and specialized internships were the status internships. Specialized internships were essentially the first year of residency in whatever the chosen specialty was. Each of us saw the Dean of Students individually to discuss our plans for post-graduate placements.

He was not at all happy with my choice of a rotating internship. As a member of Alpha Omega Alpha, the medical honor society, I knew I was in the top 10% of my class. The dean saw me as an easy placement in a good specialized internship, so I understood his challenge of my decision. But I outlined for him my intention to get a broad final look at the rest of medicine, since I would be training in psychiatry after that. Moreover, I knew that statistically about 25 to 30% of patients in any physician's office would have psychiatric issues complicating or even causing their physical symptoms. We had a very long, 45-minute discussion about my decision to opt for a rotating internship, and he tried to talk me out of it for most of that time. I will have to hand it to him, when he finally accepted my decision, he had me placed in an excellent rotating internship at the State University of Iowa Hospital (SUIH) in Iowa City, Iowa and I will always be grateful for that. It was one of the best experiences of my training and sadly, it turned out to be the last year that SUIH offered a rotating internship. They were already developing some very strong specialized internships during the year I was there and they went with the national trend away from a more generalized training. I still believe that this was a serious mistake for medical education generally. For many of us the trade school model has always worked best and the rotating internship is an excellent opportunity to refine all your medical knowledge and skills at a higher level of responsibility so that you carry that with you into whatever your specialized practice is.

CHAPTER FOUR

Internship

I started my internship on July 1, 1966 at the State University of Iowa Hospital in Iowa City, Iowa. I had graduated from the University of Virginia Medical School in early June, 1966 and had taken the State Board Examinations. When I passed the boards, I was then licensed to practice medicine in the State of Virginia. I borrowed the money to get a car, a new Dodge Dart, which I drove to Iowa to start my internship. I was living in the house staff quarters as an intern since I was not married. Most of the interns were married and lived in apartments or had houses in the town. I had the advantage of access to the tunnels between the house staff quarters and the hospital, which was great during the winter. Iowa City was a town of about 20,000 not counting the university students. The students added roughly another 20,000 when classes were in session. It was about 1.5 miles south of Interstate 80. The Interstate speed limit was

85 during the day and 75 at night. I loved to drive and the cost of gas was cheap, around $0.40/gal. Instead of returning to my staff quarters, I would drive on the interstate when I got off work as driving gave me a chance to think through the issues of the day and unwind a bit before I went back to my room.

I was on call usually every 4thth night for most of my rotations. The way the schedule worked, I would be on full call every 4thth night, and every 2ndnd day I would be on call just for admissions. Once I had finished the work-up on all my new admissions, I could leave for the rest of the night. So the call schedule was not bad compared to a lot of the other internships.

The intern group was comprised of a mix of straight interns and rotating interns. By the third or fourth month, the specialized interns were more knowledgeable about their field generally while we rotating interns were in a new field and just starting out in some ways. I didn't mind that because I was interested in adding to my knowledge of medicine in general.

They fed us well at the hospital. We had the usual three meals a day and then we had midnight supper for those of us who were on call and able to make it to the cafeteria, our clinical duties permitting. It was some of the best hospital food I've ever had. If we weren't busy on the wards, we would sometimes just sit around after eating and swap stories about our current patients or about our medical school experiences or just life in general.

We had snow from time to time in Virginia, but nothing like in Iowa. I will never forget the first big snowstorm we had that winter, when the temperatures dropped to 20 below zero. We had to use the underground tunnels that connected house staff quarters to the main hospital. One of the interns was from New Orleans and he just shook his head and said "I should have realized it would be a problem when all the bank signs had + signs on the temperature readings."

While I was at SUIH, the founder of a chiropractic school was trying to get appointed to the Board of the school of medicine. He owned two radio stations and used them to pursue his goal of getting chiropractic services reimbursed on par with other healthcare services. Obviously now that is the practice, and no one thinks much about it. Back then, the idea was quite controversial. At that time chiropractors were not highly thought of by the rest of the medical community. But this man's determination, along with others, helped change that. It is now one of the alternative medical therapies that is widely accepted.

Medicine in general was in the process of changing dramatically and it was probably easier for us to see as rotating interns, second class citizens though we were. Medicare began in 1965 and was leading to more Federal regulations for medical practitioners as a whole. And the specialty internships were all the rage. There was a strong push to require physicians and other healthcare practitioners to have continuing medical education in order to maintain their licenses, something that has become a multimillion-dollar industry today. There was also talk about requiring physicians to renew their boards every 5 to 10 years so that incompetent physicians could be weeded out or forced into additional training for maintenance of their credentials. While that may sound logical, it doesn't work out well in practice; like much of the testing done in lower levels of our educational system, the tests to pass boards are not accurately indicative of one's competence at practicing medicine. I was definitely against both of those changes as were most of the other interns.

I was fortunate enough to pass my psychiatry boards shortly before renewable boards were mandated. So I have not had to do the board exams every 10 years because my board certification does not have an expiration date, for which I have always been very grateful. It is a tremendous burden for the younger physicians, financially, as well as very time consuming. But the biggest problem is that it doesn't add much to the quality of care that is currently available to the average patient. Board testing would work, if only everyone you work with fit the protocols. In real life, you need the flexibility as well as the experience to troubleshoot for and help the 40-50% that don't fit the protocols. To practice medicine well, you synthesize what the protocols say, as well as what patients have taught you, and many other pieces of information. With board testing, all the things you learn from experience are disrespected. It forces a straightjacket on your thinking. People who know how to treat people don't need to be told how to keep up with things. It happens through your practice. And it doesn't cost $10,000. Unfortunately, re-certification is about answering the question correctly. It isn't about real medicine in real life. Right now, testing takes time and energy but doesn't add a lot to the knowledge base.

Physician burnout is more of a problem. There is no test to measure competence. Now doctors are measured by their outcomes and once again, it sounds logical on the surface. But because of the system, if someone needs a high-risk surgery, and the patient may be willing to take the risk of dying in surgery for the chance to live longer, the doctor may still refuse to do the operation, because they risk damaging their average and losing their certification. So many of these patients don't even get a shot at a high-risk surgical intervention that could be life-extending.

Re-certification is expensive and time consuming and in the end it misses the point. Nonetheless, board certification renewal has been an integral part of the transition from individualized patient care to the use of algorithms and evidence based medicine to make treatment decisions. There are still some physicians who come through their training with the ability to think through a good differential diagnosis and provide patient based care, which is still the best treatment available. But most of the physicians who were taught to do the comprehensive histories and physicals are now in their 50s and 60s and are being quietly encouraged to retire as what we can offer patients is no longer respected or valued.

While insurance companies rightly get the blame for much of what challenges good patient care, it began, as I mentioned earlier, with the federal government and Medicare. But the feds were not just picking on us. While I was in Iowa there were also federal agents chasing the Amish kids through the cornfields, trying to make them attend regular public schools. Some of those children were removed from their parents and placed in foster care for a period of time. In those cases, the parents were usually accused of child neglect. I have no idea how the issue was resolved during the short term at that time. But I have not heard of anything like that since my year in Iowa. I suspect the feds finally realized there was no realistic benefit to continuing that struggle and just let it go. Those sects were never a threat to anyone and it made no sense to me to interfere with their traditional ways of bringing up their children. There were Mennonite and Amish groups throughout the Midwest and we had similar groups in the Charlottesville area. I had seen some of them as patients as a medical student and they were always very easy to work with.

One of the women in my medical school class was African American and also my lab partner in anatomy class. Barbara was not treated any differently than Dorothy and I were by our classmates. We were the three women who graduated in our class.

Another thing that I learned about much more deeply, was the trauma that African Americans, especially in the South, suffered daily. I had a number of African American patients in Iowa and they interacted just like anyone else and I didn't think anything about it. Then one day a little, elderly black man came onto one of the wards to visit with a family member. He shuffled in with his head down, avoiding eye contact and I knew immediately that he was from somewhere in the South. The contrast between him and the African American patients I was accustomed to in Iowa was very painful to see. Yet I had seen a lot of it when I was in medical school in Virginia as well as earlier in my life growing up. Dorothy, Barbara and I tried to get an apartment together when we were in medial school, but they wouldn't let us, because African Americans weren't allowed to live together. The prejudice against African Americans was so rampant, especially in the South back then. After spending 13 years in D.C. later, one of my good friends was black and became president of the Washington Psychiatric Society. He was just a very solid human being, and very good psychiatrist. As a psychiatrist, I always tried to put my patients at ease, regardless of their color or circumstances, and I treated black patients no differently. But after several months of seeing African American patients in Iowa I couldn't deny a different expectation or general shared experience between black in the Midwest and those raised in the South.

Sometime during medical school, I heard that we were considered one of the outstanding classes that apparently came along every four to five years. We were supportive of one another and everyone got along well with a few exceptions. Most of us worked hard at learning the skills necessary to become good physicians and we helped each other out when one of us was struggling. I had the same feeling with my rotating internship group in Iowa. Most of the straight interns were also a part of our group. However one or two of the straight interns were treating us as beneath them by the third or fourth month of the year. They would look down on us for not knowing as much about their specialty as they did. And, of course, we didn't know their field as well, but we did know other specialties better than they did and most of the straight interns respected that.

Internship: Obstetrics, Gynecology and Pediatrics

The State University of Iowa Hospital was the primary referral center for the medically indigent and for those with complicated or more rare medical illnesses. It was organized around the use of open wards for most patients and the wards were large, containing 24 to 30 patients in a single, large room. All the medical and surgical units were set up that way. Each unit also had 8 to 12 beds in a mix of 4-bed rooms, 2-bed rooms and private rooms that were used flexibly for patients who needed more specialized care. Some of the more severely ill patients were cancer patients who had significant immune suppression due to very aggressive chemotherapy protocols. They were in private rooms with strict isolation precautions so that they did not develop serious infections during their treatments. One of the surgical wards had a 12-bed burn unit with two 4-bed rooms, one for males and one for females. There were two private rooms and one 2-bed room. This was the only unit in the hospital where pediatric patients were in with adult patients. Gynecology was also primarily an open ward but obstetrics was organized in smaller rooms, to the best of my recollection.

I spent my first two months on obstetrics and gynecology and it was a very interesting experience. Every third night I was on call and on those nights I slept in a call room located on the unit. There was a dormitory on the grounds of the hospital where the women who were close to their due dates stayed until after their babies were born. Most of the deliveries for women who were medically indigent were done at the university hospital. There were also a few women who were at some risk of complications, or likely requiring a Caesarian section, for the safe delivery of their infants. They were also brought into the dorm earlier, so they could be monitored more closely.

I had had the chance to deliver three or four babies while I was on the obstetric rotation while I was in my fourth year of medical school. All of them involved women who had delivered other children, and the deliveries were unremarkable. Still, it is always an amazing experience to bring a new human into the world. One delivery that I chose to stay to watch was when one of the residents got to deliver his own child, under the supervision of one of the obstetric senior residents. His wife was delivering their first child and all of us there were very excited. The delivery was completely normal, the baby was a boy, and both mother and father were able to hold him for a few minutes before the nurse took him to the newborn nursery to get him cleaned up.

Most of the 20 to 25 babies I delivered during my obstetrics rotation at SUIH were routine. I was always supervised by the senior resident and the deliveries were typically done during my on call nights. I did have some patients that I saw in clinic during the day, that I was able to follow through until delivery. I also had some patients on the gynecology ward as well.

Another fascinating experience was spending three weeks in the newborn nursery. There, I was able to observe the significant differences between infants from the very beginning. Some were very easily aroused with the slightest change in their environment, such as opening the door into the nursery. Some would startle easily and would start crying almost immediately, even before they were picked up. Other babies were very laid back and didn't cry that much, even when they were getting a heel stick to get blood for lab tests. Some slept most of the time they were in the nursery, others would sleep only briefly. Some were not very active and some were squirming all over their tiny beds. We had a very small, special room for infants who were premature and this was behind the regular nursery. We had a very small infant who had weighed just over 3 pounds at birth, who was in the preemies unit. By the time I came on the unit, he weighed just over 4 pounds, and was the most active baby we had at that time. His arms and legs were long and thin and he was always in motion, except when he was asleep, which was not very often. He did not fuss or cry though. He was somewhat squirmy even when he was being held, and had been nicknamed "Spiderman" by the nurses because of his long arms and legs.

Infants who were in physical distress were treated in a small neonatal ICU on the pediatric unit. These were the babies who had respiratory distress from incompletely developed lungs at birth and were usually premature. There were also some other infants with heart defects or other congenital deformities. I did not spend time on that unit.

Many of the babies did have jaundice and had to be watched closely to make sure they did not need to have a blood exchange to bring down the concentration of bilirubin in their blood. With a significantly elevated bilirubin level, they would be at risk for cerebral palsy, with life long disability from the brain injury resulting from the toxicity of the bilirubin on the developing brain. I was able to witness one such procedure.

There were several emergency deliveries while I was on that rotation. One night one of the younger women in the dorm, started to hemorrhage bright red blood from her vagina and she was immediately rushed to the obstetrics unit for an emergency C-section. She had placenta previa, with the placenta covering the cervix, which was dilating in preparation for the baby to be born. When she started to dilate, this ruptured some of the blood vessels attaching the placenta to the uterine wall, and she was losing a lot of blood from the hemorrhaging. The nurses woke us up and we immediately scrubbed up for the surgery as she would have to go straight into surgery as soon as she got to the unit. It's amazing how fast one can go from a deep sleep into a totally alert state when the situation demands it. This was one of the most urgent obstetrical emergencies I experienced and there was no technology available at that time to forewarn us of the situation. It can be readily identified now well in advance, with the ultrasounds that are done routinely at least twice during pre-natal care. I was second assistant for the surgery and the senior resident did an excellent job of delivering the baby very quickly, so he could be given oxygen to bring him out of his cyanosis. The mother was in shock when she arrived on the unit and was immediately started on two units of blood to bring her out of the shock. Both mother and baby survived, and went home within 2 weeks. This was her first pregnancy and it was unclear whether she would be able to have another pregnancy safely.

Another woman, who had had a very difficult delivery and one that I was not present for, had given birth to her fifth child and this wasn't the first time she had had a difficult pregnancy and delivery. She and her husband were both devout Catholics and did not believe in birth control. One of the senior residents, who was also Catholic, was aware of her situation and the significant risk to her life if she became pregnant again, and he volunteered to talk with her about using some form of birth control to prevent another pregnancy. He spent some time with her, pointing out the risk for the whole family if she did not survive to care for the five children that she already had. He shared with her that he was Catholic and recognized that what he was recommending was not what the church would approve of. But he felt strongly enough about the religious dilemma she had, that he made the recommendation that she do whatever she needed to do to prevent another pregnancy. It was unclear when she left the hospital whether she would follow his recommendation, but it was clear that she was grateful for his advice, since he understood how this would be against church doctrine, and she was thinking about the decision when she was discharged. I continue to have enormous respect for the resident for his intervention with that patient and his respect for her situation. He basically acknowledged to her that both of them would be acting against the church's laws; he was in violation for recommending birth control and she would be if she followed his recommendation to prevent additional pregnancies.

I was in the process of delivering a baby one night and when I had his head out I was unable to pull him out naturally. The senior resident immediately had me give him control of the head and step back so he could do the delivery. He also had difficulty with the delivery, since the baby's shoulders were broader than his head, which is unusual. He was able to deliver him safely, but he broke the child's collarbone in order to get him out. Once he was out and we had him on the examining table we realized he was a dwarf, with the short arms and legs and the normal size torso and head. His mother looked at him and said "He's a dwarf, like his father." This was her third child and she was not unhappy that he was a dwarf. She was anxious to tell her husband about the baby and he was allowed to come into the recovery room with her. She told me later that she had another son who was also a dwarf. They had had a second son, who was not, but he had died before he was three years of age from a congenital heart defect, for which there was no available treatment at that time. She said that she would rather have a healthy dwarf than another child who was not a dwarf but had other, more serious problems. They appeared to be a close-knit family and were coping well with the dwarfism issue. This is the genetically dominant condition that actor Peter Dinkledge of *Game of Thrones* has had life long. In that TV series he brings a very poignant character to life, who does not have anything like a loving family to accept who he is.

The most interesting patient I saw while interning in obstetrics was a woman who was sent to us at about seven months into the pregnancy, which was her initial pre-natal care. I was the first to examine her and her belly felt like she had a lot of tennis balls in her abdomen. I called the senior resident over and told him I thought she was carrying more than one baby. He laughed, since I had not been on the service very long, and told me that I was likely feeling feet or elbows. Then he examined her, nodded his head respectfully in my direction, and said, "I believe you're right. It's probably twins." Hearing his conclusion, the woman said, "Oh, no! I have three other children at home and the oldest is only three." She was very upset at the thought of twins. We sent her for an X-ray, and it turned out not to be twins, but triplets. She was just stunned at the news. She was admitted to the dorm so she could be closely monitored for the duration of the pregnancy.

I was on call the night she delivered. She was still in the seventh month of the pregnancy and there was an attempt to stop her labor with IV alcohol. Apparently this had been used successfully to stop labor in other similar situations. That seems really primitive now with the options we have available today to counter pre-term labor.

Unfortunately for her, the alcohol didn't work, and she was drunk by the time she was taken to the delivery room. And she was not a happy drunk. She could not be given any additional medications for pain due to the risk this posed for the babies. She swore and cussed all of us throughout the delivery. The senior resident delivered the babies and the attending obstetrician on call supervised the deliveries. The pediatric service had been notified of the impending births of premature triplets and there were three pediatricians, two senior residents and one attending, standing to the side with three pediatric nurses, all of them ready to take the babies as soon as they were delivered. As it turned out, the babies did very well, all without significant respiratory distress, and they all weighed more than had been expected. The boy was over 4 pounds and the smallest girl was 3 pounds, 6 ounces. As each baby was delivered, a nurse would step forward to take it and she and one of the pediatricians would take the baby to one of the nearby tables to work on getting the infant evaluated and stabilized. All three babies went into the preemie nursery and none of them were on oxygen for more than 24 hours. The mother was discharged home with the boy, who had gained up to 5 1/2 pounds by the time she was ready to be released. She and her husband came back about two to three weeks later to take the older girl home when she had gained enough weight to be ready to go. The younger girl was just under 5 pounds. The parents insisted on taking both girls on that day and they were allowed to sign the younger one out AMA (against medical advice). Both parents were in their early twenties and barely making it financially before she had the triplets. All of us were concerned about how they would manage with six children under the age of four. They lived several hours away in the western part of the state and we knew nothing about their circumstances, including whether there were members of their extended families who could support them in the care of all the children. All we could do was hope they did have support at home.

Within a few more days, I finished the first two-month rotation on obstetrics and gynecology and was on to the second two-month rotation on pediatrics.

The pediatric unit was also the referral center for medically indigent children who were seriously ill. It was also the main unit to treat children with cancer. Most of the children on the unit had cancer and one of the attending physicians, (we called them "attendings") Dr. Lescarij, was the pediatric oncologist who worked closely with the other oncologists treating the adult cancer patients. While I don't remember if I'm spelling Dr. Lescarij's name correctly, he was an excellent teacher and made no distinctions between those of us who were rotating interns and those who were straight pediatric interns.

He would get an admission of a child brought in for treatment of cancer and one of us interns would be assigned to the patient. We would do an admission history and physical exam and he would then go over our findings and discuss the examination and our diagnostic impressions with us. These discussions were done mostly in the chart room behind the nurses station, but would occasionally take place at the bedside, sometimes with the parents present and sometimes not. If the diagnosis of cancer had already been made by the referring physician, he would usually see the parents privately after we had gone over the initial findings.

He told me that if he was the one who first told them that their child had cancer, he would go over very briefly with them the type of cancer and the likely treatment options, answer any questions they had and then schedule a time to see them the next morning for a more thorough discussion of their child's diagnosis and treatment. He said that he knew the parents wouldn't be able to remember anything else he said after he told them that their child had cancer. He would give them a prescription for a sedative so they could get some sleep overnight, and then send them back to wherever they were staying. The next morning the parents had had time to take in the diagnosis and were better able to discuss the implications of the diagnosis and to take part in the planning for their child's treatment.

The parents were not allowed to stay with their children during the night. Visiting hours were limited throughout the hospital to a few hours during the afternoon with somewhat longer hours on the weekends. The rule was that all visitors had to be 12 years or older. This was frequently fudged a bit, especially on weekends. Most of the patients lived several hours away and the families were not able to visit during the week anyway. Dr Lescarij allowed the mothers of his patients to remain on the unit during the day, for the emotional support of their children, who were undergoing treatments that made them very sick and were sometimes painful. The children needed the closeness with their mother after these treatments, and the mothers were very anxious to be with their children as much as possible. Dr. Lescarij understood this. He also knew that they would be better support for their children if they had time away from the unit after 8PM, to be able to focus on something else for a short while, and then get a reasonable night's rest. He was aware that they could become overwhelmed and maybe breakdown in front of the children and the other mothers, which would demoralize everyone, especially the children. They were with their children on this basis for weeks and months on end. They talked a lot to each other, both during the day with the children, and obviously also at night in the dorm. They were a tight-knit group and very supportive of each other. They still looked tired and anxious most of the time, but I did not see any of them breakdown inappropriately or create a difficult situation.

The nurses on the unit were exceptional, and also provided individual support for any of the mothers when they needed it. The most difficult situations occurred when one of the children was dying and the parents were not allowed to stay with the child if they died during the night. There was no way to tell exactly when a child would die and the usual arrangement of the parent with the child during the day and in the dorm or another appropriate local arrangement remained the rule. I was uncomfortable with this when a child was dying, but this was three or four years before Elisabeth Kubler-Ross's landmark book, *On Death & Dying* was published. Her book prompted a major and much needed rethinking and reworking of the management of terminally ill patients and their families. Now families are able to remain with the dying patient for as long as they want.

There was a four-bed unit for children with cancer, who were three years old or younger. There was a similar four-bed unit for children with other illnesses. The rest of the unit was a combination of two-bed rooms and a few private rooms. These were used flexibly as in the other parts of the hospital. Sometimes the private rooms were used for a child that was dying, but this was not always the case. This seemed to be something that the nurses would decide, depending on what seemed best for the patient and their family.

My first patient with Dr. Lescarij was a 7-year-old boy with leukemia. He was adopted and was his parents' only child. He had been sent to the university hospital for further evaluation by his primary care physician (PCP) and the parents were not initially aware of the diagnosis. He was not feeling well but was still fairly active and talkative. I did not sit in on Dr. Lescarij's discussion with his parents late that afternoon, but his blood work confirmed a diagnosis of acute leukemia and he was going to need chemotherapy. Five year survival rates for almost all the cancers were still not very good, but there was still a slim chance of survival with some of the treatments that were then available. His discussion with the parents did not go well and the boy's mother left abruptly, quickly followed by his father. When they returned the following morning they demanded to take him out of the hospital. His mother was very insistent that this could not be an accurate diagnosis and she was going to seek out a better evaluation. Dr. Lescarij listened to her concerns and, when it was clear that she could not accept the diagnosis, he gave the parents suggestions of other medical centers where their son could also get excellent care. He did not make them sign him out AMA (against medical advice) and wrote the discharge order at the end of his discussion with the parents. I asked him why he was not more insistent with them and he told me that he had seen other parents with this reaction and knew that they would eventually have to accept the diagnosis as the boy became worse. It was his hope that once they accepted the diagnosis, they would allow the boy to have the treatment that he needed and would be able to work appropriately with whichever cancer center they felt most comfortable with. He had also left it open for them to return to his service for their son's treatment if they chose to. He said that sometimes they would return, but many times they did not.

Amy

One of my patients was a young girl, whom I shall call Amy, and her story was one of the most important and compelling experiences during my training. Amy was 9 or 10 years old and she was referred to the university hospital with a diagnosis of possible leukemia. She had a white count over 100,000 in a complete blood count (CBC) done by her pediatrician, who had made the referral. The parents had been informed that it was very likely that she had some form of leukemia. She was one of the middle children in a large Iowa farm family. She had five or six siblings. The family was a close one and they were all hoping that they would get better news from the staff at the university hospital.

Amy had been in good health until about three weeks prior to her admission. The first indication that something was wrong was significant bleeding from her gums when she brushed her teeth. Within a few days she reported not feeling well, feeling tired and fatigued all the time, in spite of sleeping longer than usual. She began to have bruising under the skin with even minor pressure on the skin. They took her to the pediatrician who examined her and found enlargement of the liver and spleen in addition to the other problems she had presented with. He did the CBC which showed a very high white count. The normal white blood cell count is between 4000 and 10,000. He knew the most likely diagnosis was leukemia and he sent her immediately to us.

She was one of the patients assigned to me and I did the initial history and physical. She clearly did not feel well and her mother did most of the talking. She described Amy as a lively, smart and very talkative child before her illness. She was very worried about her daughter and Amy did not want her to leave her side. The child was anxious about being in the hospital, but mostly she wanted her mother with her because she felt bad. On the physical exam, she had bruising and small, petichial hemorrhages over most of her body. (Petichial hemorrhages are small red or purple spots on the skin, indicating a minor bleed from broken capillary blood vessels.) When I looked in her eyes with the ophthalmoscope, the optic nerve appeared normal, which meant that it was unlikely that she had increased pressure on the brain. She responded briefly, but normally to questions I asked her as I was doing the physical exam. There were no neurological abnormalities on the initial exam. She complained of pain and tenderness when I examined her abdomen. I could feel the enlargement of both the spleen on her left side and the liver on her right side. Her heart and lungs appeared normal. She had already had blood work drawn and it was sent to the lab to be done stat.

Dr. Lescarij came in as I was finishing up and he did a quick exam of the abnormal areas. He then asked her mother to come to his office to talk with her about the diagnosis and treatment. One of the nurses stayed with her to help her get adjusted to the unit. We went to his office and as gently as he could, he told her that Amy did have leukemia and that it was a particularly severe case. The lab work was back and her white count was just under 200,000. He diagnosed her with acute myloblastic leukemia, which was involving primarily the granulocytes, one of the types of white blood cells. He discussed with her mother the importance of getting treatment started quickly and he told her Amy would be receiving very aggressive chemotherapy medications, starting the next day. He told her that Amy would feel very sick from the medicines and that they would do their best to make her as comfortable as possible. He did tell her that she would lose her hair for the duration of the treatments.

Amy's mother had clearly been expecting bad news. But she was overcome for several minutes as she realized that her daughter's chances of survival were very low. Dr. Lescarij talked with her about how unusual Amy's case was and that they were going to use an experimental protocol since this leukemia was very invasive. Her mother signed the necessary permissions for her daughter's treatment and she asked about staying with Amy during the hospitalization. Dr. Lescarij let her know about the rule regarding visitation and that she would not be able to be with Amy during the night, so that she, the mother, could get some rest in order to be of help to her daughter during the day. She accepted this and indicated she would make arrangements for a place to stay. She was told about the dorm and was somewhat relieved that that was available. She indicated that she was going to talk with her husband and he would join them as soon as he could make arrangements for someone to take over the necessary farm work. She was given a prescription for a sedative but was not sure that she would use it. Dr. Lescarij let her know that that was her decision, but he wanted her and her husband to have it available if they needed it. She then left and returned to Amy's room.

Blood work was drawn the next morning and the treatments were started. Her white count was over 300,000 that morning. She was very sick with the treatment and was throwing up most of the day. She had some diarrhea, but this was not as much of a problem as the vomiting, as she had not eaten much for the previous several days. She was restless and uncomfortable throughout that first day, but was a little better the next day. As I recall, she was to have the treatments on a weekly basis, so we expected that she would gradually improve until the next treatment, especially if she had a good response to the treatment. We were hopeful that the white count would decrease to closer to normal, hopefully under 50,000. She seemed to feel a little better for two or three days, and then began to feel worse again. She did not get the large decrease in her white count we had hoped to see. It did drop from over 300,000 down to 150,000 over the first three days following the treatments, but then it began to increase again.

On the fourth day after the treatment, she clearly was taking a turn for the worse. Her white count that morning was over 250,000 and was increasing rapidly. She was sleeping most of the time and was becoming difficult to arouse. She was irritable when she was awake and her mother said that she had never seen her like this before. It was the weekend and some of her older siblings were at the hospital and having short visits with her. Her father had returned home after a short visit with Amy, to deal with the farm work, since this was harvest time and most of their neighbors were too busy with their own farms to provide the needed help at Amy's family's farm. Her siblings were to stay with their mother for a few days, until their father could make another visit to Amy and then take them home.

By the end of the afternoon, it was clear that she was losing ground rapidly. Dr. Lescarij was in to see her during the early evening and he could barely arouse her. Her mother had taken the other children to get something to eat and was not there when he made rounds. He ordered another CBC before he left. I was on call that night and he told me to call him as soon as the results came back, no matter what time it was. He also told me to check her one more time before I went to bed and let him know what her status was at that point.

I was busy that night and did not get back to check her until almost 11. I had instructed the nurses to inform me if they noticed a significant change in her and they had monitored her closely throughout the evening. She had had a slow decline over the evening and they knew I would be checking her again once the other work was done. Almost as soon as I was back to check her, we got her CBC results. Her white count was over 600,000. When I looked into her eyes I could not see anything recognizable. There were a lot of dark areas and some smaller white areas. I could not see the optic nerve at all. I could not arouse her and she made small grimaces of pain when I tried.

When I got back to the chart room, I immediately called Dr. Lescarij and told him that I couldn't arouse her and I told him that her white count was over 600,000. He said, "I'll be there in 20 minutes." I was stunned. I had never seen an attending come in when he was not on call. I was anxious that perhaps I should have called him sooner, even though we did not yet have the white count. He asked me about the optic nerve and I had to tell him that I could not even see it, but did not know how to describe what I did see. He said he would take a look at it when he got there.

I talked with the nurses while I waited for him to get to the hospital. They were doing the report for the shift change and I frequently sat in on that when I was on call, so that I could be aware of any problems that might come up during the night. So they were used to me being there. They reassured me that Dr. Lescarij usually came in when one of his patients was likely to die overnight and that they had already guessed that Amy would be one of those patients. They also told me that her mother and siblings were out in the lobby area of the hospital and wanted to talk with me if possible, before I went to bed.

When he arrived, we went back to Amy's room, and began to examine her. He was unable to arouse her either. He looked in her eyes with the ophthalmoscope and just shook his head. He then had me look into her eyes again. He explained that what I was seeing was bleeding into the eye with the dark areas being very thick blood and the white areas being where the serum had separated out from the blood. He then said, "The bleeding you see in the eye, is also going on in the brain. There is very likely pressure building up in the brain, from all the bleeding in the enclosed space of the skull and we have no way of stopping it." He asked if I knew how to contact her mother and I told him that she was in the lobby of the hospital, waiting to hear something about Amy's condition. He then told me to come with him while he talked with her.

We went out to the lobby and she was sitting there, anxiously awaiting to know what was happening with her daughter. There were 3 or 4 of her siblings in other chairs in the lobby. They were very quiet, but all were awake and wanting to know what we could tell them. Dr. Lescarij took her mother aside, to give us some privacy, and told her as gently as he could that Amy would likely die within the next one to two days, possibly even during this night. He told her that Amy's white count was higher than it had been at any time since she entered the hospital. He also told her that she had bleeding in the brain and was in a coma. He said she did not appear to be suffering, but that there was no hope that she could recover from this. Her mother broke down and cried for several minutes, and then asked if she and the other children could stay in the lobby for the rest of the night so they could at least be that close to her. He told her that he would let the nurses know that they would be there and that she would be informed if anything changed with her daughter. He told her that I was on call for the night and I would keep her informed throughout the night if anything changed.

He then went back with me to the unit and we went into the chart room. He had us sit down and he made a short note in her chart. He then told me to have the nurses wake me every two hours so I could go in and examine Amy to see if anything had changed. He told me that it was very likely that she would die that night, but this could go on longer as he had told her mother. He told me to talk to her mother about how Amy was doing or if things remained unchanged. She clearly wanted to be with her daughter for the last time that she had and I was very sorry that she was not allowed that. As I have mentioned earlier, this was before Elisabeth Kubler-Ross's book was published and the issues of death and dying became widely known, leading to changes in how these situations were managed.

The last thing Dr. Lescarij talked with me about before he left, was how to get permission from her mother for an autopsy. Autopsies were done much more frequently at that time, but we both knew that her mother would have a hard time giving permission for the autopsy. He talked about how important it would be in a case like this and how important the findings could be for additional research into this unusual form of leukemia. He ended by saying that I should be present for the autopsy, if we had permission, and it would likely be around 10 in the morning if she died during the night. He asked if I had any questions and when I didn't, he left and returned home.

It was after one a.m. and I went back to check her one more time. I then told the nurses to wake me at 3, 5 and 7 for checks on her and to talk with the family. I then went to the call room on the unit and went to sleep. By then I had mastered the art of falling asleep quickly when I was on call, especially knowing that I was likely to be called out again before the night was over. I was waked up for the checks at 3 and 5. She seemed to be stable but unresponsive at those checks and I then went out to talk briefly with her mother. The other children were still there but some of them had arranged the chairs so that they could sleep. Her mother was never asleep when I came to talk with her and I know she did not sleep at all that night.

One of the nurses came and woke me at about 6:10 and I knew what she was going to tell me. She said that Amy had passed away a few minutes ago. I went and checked her and pronounced her dead as of 6:14 a.m. Then I went out to talk with her mother and told her that she had died without ever waking up and that she had died quietly and in no distress. She broke down and cried hard for several minutes and I held her hand and just let her cry. I took her to the same area where Dr. Lescarij and I had talked with her the previous night and talked with her about the importance of doing an autopsy as soon as possible. I explained the importance for research of the findings in a rare case like Amy's and that it was one of the ways new and better treatments for childhood leukemia could be developed to help other children like Amy.

It was clear that she was very conflicted about it. She asked if she could see her one last time while she was still on the unit, and I said I would arrange it for her. She agreed to sign consent for the autopsy. I took her back with me to the unit and had one of the nurses take her to see her daughter. Amy looked very much as she had the evening before when her mother had seen her last. The nurse stayed with her until she was ready to leave and then brought her to me. She was still tearful but she went ahead and signed the consent form for the autopsy. I told her how sorry I was that we had not been able to save her daughter and she gave me a quick hug before leaving the unit and going back to her other children.

Dr. Lescarij and I met in the autopsy room at 10:00 a.m. We stood across from the pathologist who would do the autopsy. It felt very strange to see Amy there. I could easily remember how she had been when she first entered the hospital and all of that was now gone. I watched as the pathologist opened the chest and abdomen. She had also had significant bleeding in the abdominal organs, and both the spleen and liver were substantially larger than normal. The pathologist and Dr. Lescarij talked about all the abnormal findings and showed me the signs of her illness that were fairly unique. When he opened the skull, there was a lot of bleeding intracranially and both said there was no way that was survivable. I don't remember the details of all that they showed me, but it was a profound experience to see this child dead and being autopsied. I had only seen two autopsies in medical school. This is the only one for someone I had known prior to their death.

As I said when I began this story, this was one of the most important experiences in my medical training. I was very sad to see this little girl die in such a short time. But I was also profoundly impressed at seeing Dr. Lescarij come back to the hospital that night and show me, by his example, how to deal with a patient and the family when the patient was eminently terminal. It was exceptional mentoring. My ability to deal with similar situations throughout my medical career is really due to what he taught me that night.

There is nothing that will spare you the anxiety of having to make decisions regarding life and death issues in your patients. However, having a well thought-out approach to dealing with these times in a comforting and compassionate way was a gift that I have always carried with me since that night. He taught me by example, around the care of one of our patients, and I have been able to draw on that experience many times in the years that followed. This is one of the most important aspects of being a physician and one that is most difficult to teach in any other way than the way that Dr. Lescarij showed me that night. It has been truly invaluable and I have been forever grateful to him for the thoughtfulness and compassion with which he helped all of us on that painful and difficult night.

Becky

One of the other, really tragic patients that I saw on pediatrics, was a nine month old baby girl who was sent in by one of the pediatricians in a rural, outlying county, unaccompanied by any family members. I will call her Becky. She was admitted with severe dehydration, secondary to severe diarrhea. The court in the county of origin was apparently investigating the family for severe neglect of this infant and the possibility that the child was the product of incest from the father sexually abusing the baby's mother, his daughter, who was 16 at the time the child was born. There were younger children in the home and apparently the mother was deceased. The father was the only parent in the home for some time before this child was conceived. She had been full term at birth with a birth weight of 7 to 8 pounds. When she arrived on the unit she weighed 9 pounds and was 9 months old. She was dehydrated and would have weighed 1 to 3 pounds heavier without that. However it was very clear that she was severely malnourished and had gained very little weight following her birth, secondary to the severe neglect, which included actual starvation for this child.

She was critically ill when she arrived and we had to immobilize her so that we could get IVs started to treat the dehydration. We also had to take blood for basic lab work and we sent specimens of the diarrhea and of her urine, as soon as we could get that specimen, for stat results on the cause of her diarrhea and the status of her other organs. She actively avoided eye contact with any of the staff, turning her head away from us as far as she could turn it. She made a continuous crying noise that sounded as if she was frightened and/or in pain, but made no other verbal sounds. Initially, she could not be comforted and seemed to respond to any attempt to make a soothing contact with her as if she was fearful that we would hurt her. Once we had the IV going and the diarrhea under some level of control, she curled up in the crib in a fetal position and she also hid her face against the end of the crib. She continued to make the crying sound, but it was softer once no one was touching her or coming too close to the crib. The sound appeared to be an attempt at self-soothing. She did not look around for anyone to take care of her and clearly did not expect any kind of comfort or soothing from any of us. The nurses were very worried about her because of this, fearing that she might be mentally retarded, because of her lack of emotional connection with any of her caretakers.

Over the next few days, as she got somewhat acclimated to her new situation, she began to show some response to the nurses who were taking care of her the most, showing less fear and anxiety with them. She also would go for longer periods of time without making the continuous crying sound she had made initially. She still cried with diaper changes because her bottom had been severely inflamed from the diarrhea and she had likely not had diapers changed frequently while she was still with her biological family. She was beginning to eat some baby food and was also taking frequent bottles of formula. She began to gain weight and she was developing a good appetite. She began to tolerate having one of the nurses hold her when giving her a bottle and seemed to be beginning to enjoy that experience. She was still not verbal and did not do any of the babbling that babies her age normally do as part of their learning to talk. I rotated off of pediatrics after about 10 days, so I did not follow her development after that.

However, I did see her again about 6 months later. I had gone back to the pediatric unit to follow up on a child who had had surgery for a biopsy of an early childhood tumor, prior to starting chemotherapy. As I finished with that child, one of the nurses came to get me to come to the nurses station to see Becky, who was still on the unit. By this time she appeared to be a normal weight for her age of 15 or 16 months. One of the nurses was carrying her on her hip and I learned that they carried her around most of the day, taking turns with who had her at any given time. She was beginning to talk and was clearly attached to the nurses who had been her caregivers for the past 6 to 7 months. She was apparently going to continue to reside on the unit for an indefinite period of time, as the department of social services did not yet know what placement to arrange for her. She appeared to be thriving with all the attention and care she was getting on the unit and she was making good progress in catching up on her developmental milestones, though she was still somewhat behind her age mates in some areas. She appeared to be interacting with the nurses in a normal way and I was enjoying seeing her interactions with them. The nurses were talking about how happy she was and she was clearly the pet of the unit. I was talking with the nurses about her progress and after a few minutes she appeared to notice my presence, and that I was someone new. She then looked at me with a big smile on her face. And my heart sank. Because there was an emptiness in her eyes, similar to what I had seen previously in chronically schizophrenic or psychotic psychiatric patients. And I knew that the damage from her severe neglect was still very much an issue. I made a rapid decision not to voice these concerns, as it was clear to me that she did have strong attachments to the nurses on the unit and they, better than me, could see her growing ability to attach to caring people.

But I came away from the unit with a deep sadness for that little girl, who had been so severely damaged by her biological family for the first 9 months of her life. She was making a good recovery in many ways and no longer appeared to be retarded. But I have never been able to forget the emptiness in her eyes when she smiled at me, and I have often wondered what happened to her as she got older. She was likely eventually placed with a foster and/or adoptive family and I would expect that when she was discharged from the pediatric unit, that she had a very difficult time with the transition, as this was her first experience of being cared for by people who genuinely loved her and were not dangerous and neglectful, the way her biological family had been. I hope that she was able to continue to be with people who genuinely cared for her. No doubt she would have had to have help during life transitions that involved losses or separations. Because I knew that she would carry vulnerabilities in those situations for the rest of her life and I could only hope that kind and understanding people would be there for her when she had to face those issues, as we all have to do in this life.

Cathy

The last case that I will discuss from my time on the pediatric unit, was a pre-teen girl whom I will call Cathy. She was about 11 years old and had been referred into the university hospital for a full evaluation, since she had some learning difficulties and was falling further behind her age mates in terms of her social maturation. She had been overweight all of her life and her parents had tried multiple diets with her, without success. She did not get along well with her peers and would become irritable and difficult to manage when she did not get her way. She was also noted to have frequent staring spells and was to be evaluated for a possible seizure disorder or other neurological problem. She wore very thick glasses, but was continuing to complain of problems with seeing things clearly. Routine eye testing did not disclose any problems with her eyes, that her glasses could not have compensated for, but she continued to complain that she was not seeing well. She was in special education classes and her grades had been falling in recent months. I got an ophthalmology consult as well as a neurology consult for further evaluation of her visual problems as well as the possibility of seizures. She had no evidence of seizures on the EEG and no abnormal neurologic findings. Her initial ophthalmology evaluation was unremarkable.

She was immature for her age. She was also in early puberty with beginning breast development. Her parents had asked for the evaluation so they could better plan for the remainder of her education. It was clear that her parents were hoping for better results on her IQ testing. They were very disappointed that she continued to test out in the mildly mentally retarded range.

They had noted that she seemed more clumsy in recent months, and seemed to be accident prone, with more frequent falls, which was a new development. She was more likely to run into things when she was walking, even at her home that she was very familiar with. I put in a second ophthalmology consult, specifically asking to have her tested for problems with depth perception. Again, they found no evidence of abnormal depth perception in the second evaluation.

I went in to see her again after that report, as she did seem to have difficulty with accurately distinguishing various objects around her. I noticed her tentatively reaching out toward objects that she could see, but would have to feel around before she could touch the object and then she could pick it up. On impulse, I showed her a quarter I had pulled out of my pocket and asked if she could see it. She said she could see it, but again she groped toward it before she was able to touch it and then take it into her hand. I had her give it back to me and then I tossed it onto her bed. I asked her to pick it up off the bed. She ran her hand over the bed covers in the vicinity of where she thought it had fallen. She did several broad sweeps back and forth before she finally connected with it and then she could pick it up. I then put in a third consult to ophthalmology and I talked to the senior resident on ophthalmology, describing what I had seen her do when she was trying to accurately locate objects, especially what happened when she was trying to locate the quarter I had tossed on the bed. He listened to the description and said that they would need to do an indirect examination of her retina, a procedure that was relatively new. It was difficult to do because it involved dilating her pupils as much as possible and then holding one lens in front of her eye and holding a second lens in front of the examiner's eye, lined up so that he would have a magnified view of the retina. She would have to follow his directions to look up or down or to the side, so that he would be able to see as much of the retina as possible. He arranged to have the exam done later that day and said he would call me with the results. The examination disclosed a rare, progressive disease of the retina called retinitis pigmentosa, for which there was no treatment. He said that she was going blind and would be completely blind within a few years. He said that he thought she had a rare, congenital disease that would manifest with the eye disease, mental retardation, obesity and frequently some abnormalities of sexual development, including sterility in some cases. He said he would talk with her parents to let them know what they were dealing with.

Her parents were directed to the ophthalmology department, where they met with the senior resident. He called me shortly after the meeting, to warn me that the parents were very upset and would likely take her out of the hospital. As soon as I could, I went back to Cathy's room and her parents were packing her things. Her mother said that she did not think her daughter was going blind and they were going to consult with another ophthalmologist about the diagnosis. I notified the attending pediatrician for the unit about the situation and he came in to talk further with them. I could see no reason to have them sign her out AMA, particularly since we really had no effective treatment to offer Cathy in terms of the retinal disease. Her evaluation was essentially completed and the news was worse than anything any of us expected. She would always need help as an adult, because of her blindness and her limited intellect. The attending listened to their rejection of the findings and encouraged them to seek a second opinion if that was what they wanted. He discharged her that afternoon and they left the hospital. Her mother was clearly angry and agitated. Her father didn't have a lot to say. Cathy was worried because her patents were so upset, and she clearly did not understand what had happened. I just hoped that they would follow up with someone who could work with so them, so they could begin to plan for Cathy's future in a realistic and helpful way.

CHAPTER FIVE

Internship: Adult Medicine

After finishing my pediatrics rotation, I went into four months of medicine. I had three months of ward medicine with one month of neurology as an elective. When I moved on to ward surgery, the identical ward structure was also used there. I did ward surgery for the last four months of my internship year. On medicine I had two nonconsecutive months on female medicine and one month on male medicine. Ward medicine was exactly what it sounds like. We were on 24 to 30 bed wards with rows of beds lined up on both sides of the ward, with a wide center aisle where staff could move back and forth as needed for the care of the patients. There were curtains that could be pulled around each individual bed to provide privacy when that was needed. The main nurses station was on one side of the ward as you came through the entrance. Just behind the nurses station was the chart room where physicians made their chart notes. There was an open area between the nurses station and the chart room so the charts could be quickly passed back and forth between the medical team. There was also a chart cart that we used to carry the charts as we did morning rounds on the ward. Across from the nurses station and the chart room was an exam room, used for initial physical exams and minor procedures. It also contained the crash cart (used for emergency resuscitations) and other supplies and medications for the unit. Everything was readily accessible for any emergencies on the ward, as well as any special or minor procedures that could be done on the ward. We were the primary referral center for the medically indigent for the whole state of Iowa. We were also the referral center for very complex medical problems and/or patients in need of highly specialized treatments.

Having not previously been exposed to this method of delivering medical care, I was concerned about the lack of privacy for the patients on the wards. However, within a couple of weeks, I became very impressed by the ease with which the patients could be followed by the nursing staff, who were constantly scanning the ward, looking for signs of trouble in the patients, and quickly responding to anyone who appeared in need. The patients, for the most part, did not seem to mind the lack of privacy and most patients struck up friendships with other patients and provided a lot of support and companionship for each other while they were there. They were at times the ones who first alerted medical staff to someone in need of immediate attention. Many of them stayed for several weeks, and, because of the distances involved, had only weekly visits from their family members. For the patients who were able to be up and around, they could leave the unit to go to the snack/newsstand shop if they wanted to, and they usually went in a small group. They would also bring back items for the patients who could not go, if they needed something the snack/newsstand shop carried. Visitors to the ward would usually interact with other patients and their family members during visiting hours. On the infrequent occasions, when someone on the unit was crashing, the more active patients would usually round up the visitors, especially if there were children present, and take them to the snack bar or the main lobby area, until the situation was resolved. This left the medical staff free to deal with whatever the emergency was, without worrying about the visitors. Ancillary staff, like the ones who brought up the meal trays, generally were quick to move out of our way and did not require prompting.

In addition to the ward beds, we usually had several semi-private and private rooms which were used flexibly for patients who needed isolation, or other, more specialized needs that were not appropriate for the ward environment. The call schedule for the interns was one full call night every fourth night and one evening call two days later, when we could leave the ward for the rest of the night, once all of our admission work-ups were completed and all of the other work on our regular patients was done. The medical staff on each ward consisted of one rotating intern, one straight medicine intern, two first year medical residents, a third year medical resident and an attending medical internist. All the staff would be present for morning rounds and the residents were available for any questions we had about any of our new admissions or our ongoing patients throughout the day. Morning rounds would usually take 1 1/2 to 2 hours each day and we had the rest of the day for following up on the orders and procedures developed during rounds. There were frequent discussions about the differential diagnoses of new patients and we were all expected to be able to formulate a reasonable differential diagnosis and to be able to demonstrate the relevant physical findings on each of our patients. Thinking through each patient's diagnosis and relevant lab tests and procedures, and being able to describe how all this information could be used to confirm or change the diagnosis, was something we were expected to do routinely. It was a hard discipline to maintain but it became the bedrock of my approach to all my patients' medical issues.

My second rotation on medicine was a rotation on neurology, where I followed the residents around and had very limited responsibility for direct patient care. I was not on call that month, which was a welcome break for me. I saw a lot of interesting patients while I was on neurology. There were two or three patients with long-standing seizure disorders, who were also having hysterical seizures as well.

One had what looked like a focal motor seizure, with continuous jerking movements of her right hand and forearm. However, there was no evidence on the EEG of any changes since the prior EEGs done for follow-up of her grand mal seizure disorder. And her seizures appeared to be well controlled with her current doses of anti-convulsant medications.

She was experiencing a lot of situational stress, and was low functioning for the most part. Her boyfriend recently broke off their relationship. She had only a sixth grade education, and she couldn't keep a job. Currently, she was still dependent on her parents. When she was observed while asleep, she no longer had significant jerking movements, but if she was aroused at all the jerking movements would start again. Since by then all of the house staff knew that I was going into psychiatry, the residents suggested that I talk with the patient and her parents about her situation.

I agreed and I let the patient and her parents know that this was not a new seizure disorder and that her medications for her grand mal seizure disorder were still giving her good seizure control. They did not need to be changed. Community mental health centers were becoming more widely available and I suggested that they see if there was a program in their home county where she could get into a day treatment program or a sheltered workshop so that she had a supportive program that she could take part in during the week. I also suggested she be evaluated by a psychiatrist to see if medication might be helpful in managing her anxiety symptoms. They were agreeable to trying that and we set up a psychiatric consultation for her prior to her discharge, informing the consulting psychiatrist that she could possibly benefit from whatever services were available in her home county.

I also saw some patients with brain tumors at different stages of that process, from initial diagnosis to terminal care. There was a wide range of symptoms in these patients, from localized neurological signs to personality changes to the initial onset of seizures secondary to the tumor.

I was able to see new patients in the neurology clinic and I was able to diagnose a woman with Huntington's chorea. Huntington's chorea is a genetic neurological disease that is autosomal dominate, meaning that statistically 50% of the offspring of an affected individual will have the disease. Its onset is usually in middle age, around the 40s or 50s. She had the early involuntary movements which she tried to mask by completing them as voluntary gestures. She had been a teacher and was worried that the movements might be Huntington's. She told me that she had a younger sister who was diagnosed with Huntington's and was currently in a nursing home with the dementia that can be part of the Huntington's syndrome. She had been referred to the clinic to evaluate the possibility that she had the disease. She had been hoping that, since she did not have symptoms when her sister was diagnosed, that she would not get it. Sadly, she did have the disease and was admitted for a full evaluation. I talked with the resident on the clinic that day and asked if there was anything available in the way of treatment for Huntington's and he indicated that we did not have any effective treatments at that time. I had actually seen a young woman with Huntington's chorea on one of the back wards at Western State Hospital in Staunton, Virginia while I was in medical school. This was during one of the class visits to the state hospital, so that we would know what that was like, similar to the trip we took to the Lynchburg colony during my third year of medical school. This patient had had an unusually early onset of the illness and was 25 years old when I saw her in the hospital. She was tied into her hospital bed to keep the severe jerks from throwing her out of the bed. She had had numerous fractures from the severe involuntary jerking movements throwing her out of her bed or causing serious falls when they occurred earlier in the course of her illness. She had some dementia at the time we saw her. She was heavily sedated to make her as comfortable as possible with the confinement to her bed and the continuous restraints. Both the neurology resident and I knew that this patient did not have a good prognosis and she had come, partly hoping that she would get a diagnosis of something more benign than the Huntington's, which was now surfacing. And we really had nothing to offer her in the way of hope, because the illness is one that is relentlessly progressive. It is now possible to do genetic testing to determine if an individual carries the gene responsible for Huntington's. Because the affected individuals are in their 40s and 50s, they generally already have children who carry the gene and are subject to the disease later on. Prevention is more in the decisions the children of these individuals make in terms of whether to have their own biological children. There is no cure for the disease, but there are some beneficial treatments with medicines used in psychiatry and neurology that can lesson some of the symptoms.

Andrew

My third month of adult medicine was male medicine, where I encountered a very difficult patient, a young man I'll call Andrew. He was a young man in his late twenties with an extremely fast moving lung cancer. He was in one of the private rooms on the unit, because he was on a very aggressive medication protocol, and was at risk for significant immune suppression. I inherited him from the intern who was taking care of him on the service before we moved to our next rotations. He filled me in on the details of his treatment over the past two months in the hospital. He had been diagnosed with an oat cell cancer of the lungs, which was inoperable, and he was currently failing the first protocol of anti-cancer medicines that he was taking. He was married and his wife was staying close by and was with him every day. His parents also visited frequently. All of them were very supportive of him and they were very concerned about the aggressive and lethal nature of his tumor. The intern went over the physical findings with me and they were horrifying.

If you want to know how to visualize the size of his cancer, put your right hand, palm down, along the right side of your stomach, where you can feel the top of the hip bone. Place your left hand, also palm down against your upper right chest just over the right collarbone. That accurately measures the length of the tumor. Then take your left hand, pointing straight up, and place it about two inches to the left of your breastbone. From there to the outer chest wall on the right side is the width of the tumor. The cancer was pushing his left lung and his heart into his left chest wall. He was on full oxygen because his breathing was so compromised. He had cancer in his liver, which normally lies under the lowest ribs under the right chest and there was no way of identifying what was left of his liver as the tumor was crowding out most of the organs in his stomach. He was on demerol for his pain every 3 to 4 hours, but he always had some level of pain and discomfort. He was withdrawn and quiet most of the time, but was always cooperative with his treatments, even though they made him very sick. He was showing some symptoms of air hunger, but was still able to talk and carry on a conversation with family or staff and was always pleasant to others, even as miserable as he was with the cancer and the chemo. He had never been a smoker and there were no familial risk factors for cancer. He had been a very productive and responsible young man prior to the onset of his cancer. All of us who knew him and treated him felt very bad for him and were hoping that he would somehow pull through.

He still maintained some hope of recovery, though he was getting more discouraged about his chances by the time I took over his care. Within a few days after coming on the service, the oncology team proposed an experimental protocol be tried in a last ditch effort to try to save his life. He was warned that his side effects might be worse, but he was willing to give it a chance. I had some concerns that it would not be effective and would just make his last days even more uncomfortable. He would be getting the treatments every three or four weeks and he had his first treatment later that same day. He had much more nausea and vomiting for the first few days but was already showing improvement in the cancer within that time. By the time he was starting to eat again, the tumor size was definitely shrinking and his breathing was starting to improve. He had been bedfast for several weeks and he began to sit up in a chair for an hour or two at a time. Soon he was going for short walks in the hall. By the second week he was able to come off the oxygen and was feeling much better. His breathing was easier and he no longer had the air hunger. He still had significant pain from the cancer, but that was also not as severe as it had been previously. He did not need the pain medicines as often, but he still required the pain medications three or four times a day. He began to talk about going home and was very anxious to do whatever was necessary to be able to go home, even if only for a few days.

At that time there were no good oral opiates available and he had been getting all of his pain medications by injection. I knew that he would need something to take by mouth if he was going to go home for a few days. So I called down to the hospital pharmacy to see if the pharmacist had any suggestions for managing his pain while at home. He asked if I had thought about methadone and I had not. I had been under the impression that it was used only with heroin addicts or for detox. The pharmacist agreed that that was the most common use of the drug. However he indicated that it also seemed to provide pain relief similar to what the injectable opiates provided and it was readily absorbed when taken by mouth. He did not have any in stock, but indicated he should be able to get a supply within one to two days. I asked him to order it and I was able to get it started the following afternoon. I talked with Andrew and his wife about using this in place of the injectable pain medications for the next 24 hours. If he had adequate pain relief with the methadone then, after several doses, I would talk with the senior resident and his attending about discharging him home either late afternoon or early the following day. They were very anxious to give it a try and it was very successful with reducing his pain, equal to if not somewhat better, than the injectable pain medication he had been taking.

By the next afternoon I had talked with the senior resident and his attending. Both had evaluated him and both were in favor of the discharge. He and his wife were ecstatic. They were both warned to keep him mostly at home, due to his immune suppression from the chemotherapy. They agreed to those terms and he was discharged home. Four days later he was brought back to the hospital because of shortness of breath, which initially seemed to be secondary to a pneumonia in his right lung. I saw him the next day on rounds and when I examined him I could feel what felt like the cancer in his abdomen and most likely in his right lung as well. He was also somewhat confused at times which was not like him at all. The residents and attending also felt he was dealing with a return of the cancer and we discussed the possibility of brain metastases to explain the change in his mental status.

His case was to be the topic of that day's Grand Rounds, a weekly meeting to present cases that were particularly difficult or were ideal for teaching both students and medical staff. The chief oncology resident presented the history of his cancer and the remarkable recovery that he had had with the experimental chemotherapy protocol. He finished his presentation by saying that they had now found the cure for this patient's cancer, and that if he died, it would be as a result of side effects of his chemotherapy, such as his current pneumonia, and not because of his cancer. I was stunned by that statement as I believed that he was still at the most risk from his cancer. I had seen enough cancer patients while in medical school, to realize that many patients who had a good response initially to their chemotherapy, did not get the same level of improvement with repeat courses of the same drug protocols. Most of them died relatively soon as a direct result of their cancer, not from the chemotherapy side effects. There are some patients that do die as a direct result of the chemotherapy, but the incidence of these is significantly lower now, with the improvements in the medications for treating cancer, and the development of medications that can treat some of the side effects more effectively.

Andrew continued to show a rapid decline over the next few days. It became clear that the tumor was back with a vengeance and, while his pneumonia improved, his breathing did not and he was back on full oxygen again. He also continued to have more problems with confusion and his mental status was clearly declining with each succeeding day. I was on call for the last day of my rotation and was concerned about his transition to a new intern the next day. He was more withdrawn and was becoming more difficult to arouse as the day went on. His wife asked to speak with me that evening and I was able to talk with her and with his parents, who were very worried about the changes in him. I talked with them about the return of the cancer and indicated that his mental status changes were most likely due to brain metastases from the cancer. They asked if he would be able to recover again with additional chemotherapy, and I told them that he would likely have a more limited response with additional chemo. His wife asked me directly if I thought he would die and

I said that I did not see any way that he would be able to live much longer. I told her how sorry I was that we were not going to be able to save him. She became very upset and ended up passing out as she was on the way back to his room. His parents called for help and one of the nurses and I were able to get her into the exam room where she could lie down until she felt better. His parents were also there with her. I told her that he might get some improvement with his next treatment, but that more than likely, he would not be able to leave the hospital again. She cried for some time and then asked what she could do for him. I told her that she and his parents had been excellent supports for him during his long hospitalization and that that had been an essential part of why he had been able to handle his illness with the courage and hope that kept him going through it all. I told them to just continue what they had been doing and the the medical team would continue his treatments as long as he showed benefit, and we would also continue to make him as comfortable as possible through the remainder of his life. He was continued on the methadone for pain once he was back in the hospital, because this did appear to give him better pain control than the injectables. When she was more in control of her feelings she thanked me for telling her what to expect and she and his parents went back to his room, where he appeared to be sleeping reasonably well. It was well past visiting hours, but I let the nurses know that they could stay with him for a while longer in view of the bad news I had just given them. I stopped in his room on my way out to the call room to sleep and let them know that I would be rotating off the service the next day, but that I would continue to get updates on his situation from the intern replacing me on the service.

I heard from the intern that he had become semi-comatose by the next day and the oncologist gave him the next treatment a few days early in an attempt to ward off his cancer a second time. He recovered enough to become conscious again for about a week and then, over a several day period, he became less and less responsive until he died quietly within the second week following his treatment. I did not get to see his wife or his parents again after that last night.

Although I had had my reservations about putting him through the experimental protocol, because it did not appear that he would live much longer, I was wrong about that. It was remarkable to see the improvement with the first course of chemotherapy. I think the most important thing that came out of that treatment was his ability to leave the hospital and have private time with his wife for the first time in months. I'm sure he also spent time with his parents and with both of their families. He even confided in me that he had been able to drive his beloved car, which I think was a Karmann Ghia, for a very short trip and he had enjoyed that immensely. That time with his wife in their own home for those four days, with other family time as he could tolerate it, his chance to drive his car for one more time and his chance to have some of his old life back for a time was the most important thing we could have given him and his family. He was sad to be back in the hospital, but very happy to have had the time with his wife for those four days. He seemed to be more accepting of his impending death, and I don't think he had any illusions about what would follow. But he appeared very grateful to have that time so he could re-experience it one last time before his death.

I was upset with the oncologist's statement during Grand Rounds, because he was so wrong about his assessment of the medicine's being a cure for this young man. Yet, I know why he said it. He wanted very much to see Andrew recover and be able to go on with his life. No one wanted to see him die. Everyone who worked with him could see his humanity, his courage and that he would have had a lot to offer, had he lived. Oncology is a very tough field to be in and I know the oncologist just wanted to give him his life back for a full life-time. We were not able to do that. But we did give him a part of his life back for those few precious days and I think that was enough for him.

Deborah

One of the most interesting patients that I had on my first rotation on female medicine was a woman that I will call Deborah. She was in her late 60s and she had been on the ward numerous times for treatment of her aplastic anemia, which was a result of her chemotherapy treatment for breast cancer two to three years previously. Aplastic anemia is the name for a condition that occurs when the body is no longer able to make blood cells, both red and white. It frequently includes the inability to make platelets as well. The only treatment at that time was transfusions every six to eight weeks. The transfusions would give her a new supply of these essential blood cells and she would then feel much better until the transfused cells decreased to the point that she had significant anemia again. The first time I saw her, she appeared weak and mildly depressed. She told me her story of the breast cancer, which continued in remission, and her need to return to the hospital every six to eight weeks for transfusions. She was anemic and she always knew when she had to return to the hospital because of how fatigued she became from the anemia. She was well known to the nurses and they immediately set her up to start the transfusions. I could tell that she had a good relationship with the nursing staff and this was also true of the medical staff as well. Her hematologist was not the attending physician for the unit that month, but he came by to see her as soon as he was notified that she was back in the hospital. She stayed in bed for most of the first two days and then she began to gradually improve over the next few days. She had a boyfriend who visited her on the weekends and it was obvious that they cared a lot about each other. I was on the ward one evening after he had just visited and she told me that she needed to be out of the hospital by the next weekend. It turned out that she and her boyfriend loved to go to the horse races and they did a little betting on the side. There was a particularly exciting horse race coming up on that weekend and she did not want to miss it. She was improved enough by the end of the week that she could be discharged by the weekend. I wished her luck on the horses as she and her boyfriend left the ward that Friday.

I saw her again about 8 weeks later, when she was back for additional transfusions. She was in better spirits that time and reported good success at the races recently. She settled into the ward, rested most of the next two days and was improving again by the end of the week. She was up and around more and she interacted with most of the patients on the unit at one time or another. Some of them she had known from previous admissions. Her boyfriend was also known to a number of the patients and to the staff as well. With that second admission, I observed her interactions with the other patients more and noted that she was somewhat of a leader with the patients once she was feeling better. We had one or two codes (patients whose hearts and/or breathing had stopped and needed immediate intervention to try to save their lives) during the time she was there and she was quick to mobilize some other patients to get visitors off the unit during such times. I also noted her ability to interact with sicker patients and help them to feel better through her upbeat attitude. I was then able to note others who also became leaders and caretakers to other, sicker patients once they were improving with their own illnesses.

By the time I was finishing my medicine rotations, I was completely won over to the ward system as an excellent and therapeutic environment for the patients. I was not aware at the time that this system was in the process of being discarded by medical authorities. There was also a similar move that had recently started in psychiatry, to close down the big state mental hospitals in favor of keeping chronically mentally ill patients in the community, rather than in institutions for the rest of their lives. The institutions were being blamed for fostering the negative symptoms that schizophrenic patients have, such as apathy, flat affect, low or no motivation and general withdrawal from the activities and people around them. For the record, schizophrenic patients are not often helped without serious medical intervention, which is best delivered and monitored in a clinical setting. Keeping anyone in their own home or community always has appeal, and is the ultimate goal, of course. But it's with misguided compassion and naiveté that we eliminated long term inpatient treatment centers for the chronically mentally ill altogether. This was another trend, in both medicine generally and psychiatry in particular, that I felt was a serious mistake.

Eleanor

There was another woman on the ward, whom I will call Eleanor, who was dying with cirrhosis of the liver. She was not my patient, but I was familiar with her from rounds and the nights when I was on call. She was very "rough around the edges." She looked like an elderly woman that you might see in some of the older western movies, but she was only in her fifties. She was a long time drinker and her cirrhosis was due to her long history of alcoholism. Her boyfriend, who visited irregularly, was also a long time drinker, and he was dressed like a typical cowboy. I can only guess that they had worked on ranches most of their lives. She was pleasant with the staff and did not make a lot of requests when she was stable. She was very ill, however, with varicose veins of the esophagus, which is a common problem with severe cirrhosis, as well as a mild chronic jaundice, due to her liver failure. She had had three episodes of severe bleeding from the veins in her esophagus. They had ruptured because of the weakened condition of the walls of the veins, which were very thin at that point. To make things worse, these veins are located in the lower esophagus, close to where it connects with the stomach, making them also susceptible to reflux of acid from the stomach, which can also be a contributing cause of the bleeding from these weakened veins.

She had been there for several weeks before I came on the ward. I had heard about the most recent episode of bleeding, which had occurred shortly after I started my rotation on that unit. She spent her days visiting with the patients who were close to her bed and, when she was not talking to the other patients, she read western novels that she clearly enjoyed. She was a bit of a fixture on the unit by that time.

After her most recent episode of bleeding, we had a lengthy discussion in the chart room, about the futility of continuing to bring her back from the brink of death, when the same bleeding episodes would continue to occur every few days, due to the weak veins in her esophagus. She had had many transfusions over the course of these episodes. We did not have the plastic intercaths at that time, to provide a less traumatic access for IVs or transfusions. PICC lines had not been developed yet. These are peripherally inserted central catheters that allow intravenous line access long term, without using a new needle and puncture to the patient with each dose of medication. Most of her veins were damaged from the previous episodes, when she was requiring IVs to maintain blood volume and transfusions to replace the blood she had lost. The attending physician as well as the house staff on the unit all agreed that she would not be resuscitated again. It would be almost impossible to find a vein that would work, and most likely she would need a cut-down to find a vein to position the needle in. They had had to resort to veins in her legs and feet with the most recent episode. Everyone agreed, including me, that there was no point in attempting to bring her back from the next episode of bleeding. Today that would be called making her DNR (do not resusitate) and this decision would be communicated to the patient and/or a close family member. But this was the 1960s; I don't know if anyone talked to Eleanor about the decision. In that time, this kind of open discussion with a patient about their impending death was generally not done, in an attempt to spare them the anxiety of knowing that they were terminal. Her boyfriend was visiting with her that day and it is possible that someone had talked to him about the situation. Since she was not my patient, I would not have been involved in those decisions and I never knew whether anyone had talked to one or both of them about there being no more resuscitations for her.

It was late afternoon, and I was the only physician on the ward, when she started to bleed again. By this time she knew when the bleeding started as she would become suddenly weak and nauseous. Apparently she had vomited blood on one or more occasions, but she was not vomiting this time. But she did know that she was bleeding out again. When she called out for help, one of the nurses came to her bedside to try to calm her. But when she did not call for medical assistance, Eleanor began to beg for help. She did want to die that day. She was crying by then and begging for help and the nurse was looking very anxious, which was unusual for any of these nurses.

I was attending one of my patients, but I quickly came to Eleanor's bedside and told the nurse to bring an IV and a cut-down tray. She brought them at once while I told Eleanor to relax, that I would most likely have to do a cut-down to get a vein, but that I should be able to start the IV quickly. Since this was the type of immediate intervention she was used to, she relaxed somewhat as I put a tourniquet on her leg and started looking for a vein. I was using a small butterfly needle, which I had used on newborns when they needed an IV, but I had no luck getting into a vein immediately. The nurse had pulled the curtains around her bed, to give her privacy, and this had been another part of the previous situations which she was familiar with. She was obviously going into shock and was very pale by then. She laid back on the pillow and watched what I was doing. I ordered the nurse to open the cut-down tray and told her I was going to make a small incision over one of the veins coming out of her foot. I told her it might hurt a little and she said that was okay. While I was doing the cut-down, the nurse was by her side telling her things would be okay soon and holding her hand to let her know that we were there for her. She became more relaxed and shut her eyes. She had a faint smile on her face as she slipped into unconsciousness. I continued to work at finding a vein for another couple of minutes and the nurse continued to hold her hand and stroke her forehead. Her breathing began to slow and within another couple of minutes, her breathing stopped. I stopped looking for a vein and moved up beside her to check for a pulse. I could not find a carotid pulse. I pulled out my stethoscope and listened for heart sounds, which were absent. I waited a few more minutes and then checked for a pulse and listened again. Both were gone and I pronounced her dead. I asked the nurse if her boyfriend was there and she said she would check. He was there and came in for a few minutes. He just stared at her, clearly not knowing what to do. I left him alone with her and he left after a few minutes. He was not crying, but did look sad and defeated.

I knew that we were not going to save her that day. She knew she didn't have much longer to live, but she did not want to die that day. I knew if I didn't start the process of getting an IV in, she would panic and I could not bear to watch her die feeling frightened and abandoned. I did not think it through before hand. I just acted to provide her with some hope and comfort as she was dying. I did not call a code, which would have brought the cardiac arrest team immediately, as I knew there was no point. So I staged a resuscitation, with the help of the nurse, and she relaxed and died with some degree of peace. Once it was over, I went back to my normal duties with my patients on the unit. No one mentioned to me anything about what I had done that day. What I did was for the patient, but also for the ward as well. It would have been very demoralizing for the patients and the nurses to watch Eleanor die, panicked and begging for help with her last breaths. I knew we couldn't save her. But I gave her what comfort I could to make her dying more manageable for her and for the rest of us. And I can't imagine that she held it against me once she had passed to the other side.

CHAPTER SIX

Internship: Surgery

I started my surgery rotations on March 1,1967, beginning with ophthalmology. I saw some of the patients who were hospitalized for surgical procedures, basically doing histories and physicals and covering any changes in their status during the day. I was not on call and also did not assist with any of the surgeries, so I was able to spend a lot more of my time in the library, as I had much more free time while on that rotation. The patients were generally immobilized for several days following their surgeries, with strict orders not to move their heads any more than necessary. No one needed to tell me how important that was — I had seen what my father had gone through when he had a detached retina following cataract surgery while I was finishing my first year of medical school. He ended up having three surgeries for the detached retina, the last two of which were done at Emory University Hospital in Atlanta. He got seriously depressed during that time, as he was unable to work and was mostly at home with nothing much to do. The inactivity was very hard for him. With that experience, I could empathize with the anxiety and depression of the patients I was following while I was on ophthalmology. I tried to be as supportive as possible, encouraging them to look ahead to being more active once they were through the first week of post-op care.

Two of the last three months of my internship, I was on general surgical wards, on call every third night, which was manageable. I spent my first month on female surgery and saw a lot of cancer patients; I was able to scrub in on some of their surgeries. Regrettably, the surgeries were frequently mutilating and many of the patients were depressed in the aftermath of treatment. Most of them were still facing chemotherapy and/or radiation as well.

By that stage of my internship, all the house staff and many of the attending physicians knew that I was going into psychiatry. Most of them were initially puzzled about why I was there. Once I had been on the unit for several days, they were aware of my interest in medicine and surgery, and they had me assist with quite a few of the surgeries. When you are an intern, assisting generally means standing across from the main surgeon, usually the senior resident, and holding retractors to keep the surgical incision open so the surgeon could perform the surgery that was needed. That is a very fatiguing thing to do, but I was fascinated with the details of the surgery and was very careful to hold the retractors so as to not interfere with the surgeon's work. After about two weeks, they accepted me as a reliable intern and they started to call on me to talk with patients who were having anxiety and/or depression and advise them of anyone who needed a psychiatric consult. By then I was a valued member of the treatment team.

One young woman in her early twenties was in follow-up care for a malignant melanoma. It had necessitated an above the knee amputation about three years earlier. They were concerned about her because she had chosen to become pregnant about 18 months prior to when I saw her. They had had concerns that she might be more susceptible to a recurrence of the melanoma because of all the hormonal changes that went with a pregnancy. She had indeed become pregnant and had an 8 month old, very active and healthy daughter at home that she clearly adored. I talked with her about why she chose to take that risk. She said that she was in a good marriage with a young man who had been very supportive of her through all the treatments. They had both wanted to have children before she was diagnosed with the melanoma. They still wanted to have children after she had completed all her treatments. They decided together that they wanted to go ahead with having a family and were going to trust God to take care of her and the baby if it was his will that they have children. She was doing very well with her prosthesis and was able to take good care of her daughter with some assistance from her husband and her mother. She had no regrets about her decision and clearly recognized the risk that she had taken. She saw the outcome as verification that she and her husband had made the right choice. Her follow-up appointment turned up no evidence of cancer and she was set up to return in six months for routine follow-up.

I saw a 16-year-old girl with a diagnosis of thyroid cancer and she and her mother were both very anxious about what this might mean. After some research that evening in the library, I learned that her thyroid cancer tended to have a better prognosis than most other cancers. When I was able to relay that information to her and her mother the next day, they were both very relieved. She had no evidence of spread and was likely facing removal of the thyroid and possible chemotherapy. She would be on thyroid medication for the rest of her life, but that would be no different than being followed up for other conditions that required life-long medications.

A more serious case was an ovarian cancer patient who was 18 or 19 years old. She had been through a very difficult course of chemotherapy, as her cancer was inoperable at the start of her treatment. Chemotherapy was initially seen as a way to extend her life, but without any hope of a cure. She had had an excellent response to the chemotherapy and the tumor was barely palpable when she returned to be re-evaluated for surgery. This was great news, but she appeared severely depressed, and I was asked to see her to talk about the surgery they were proposing. They felt they could get all of the cancer with a full hysterectomy and a radical dissection of all of the regional lymph nodes. I talked with her at length about what the surgery would be and the chance that she now had to survive the cancer. She listened to what I said, but had no questions for me, and she appeared to be almost indifferent to her situation at that point. I talked with the surgery residents and recommended that she have a psychiatric consultation as part of her work-up for the surgery. She did not indicate that she opposed the surgery. However, she did not appear to have any hope that she could recover from her cancer and I was concerned about the impact that this might have on her ability to tolerate the surgery without significant complications. I saw her just before I rotated off that service and I never knew what her outcome was.

The last patient I will discuss from the month of female surgery was a young Hispanic woman of about 19 or 20 years old. Her family was one of the migrant families that worked the farms in the mid-west. She was referred in with cervical lymphadenopathy (swelling of multiple lymph nodes in the neck) with a diagnosis of probable lymphoma. She was in no pain from the swelling and appeared healthy overall. She had had the swollen lymph nodes for several months and they were not going away. After taking the history and doing a thorough physical exam, I wrote "scrofula" as my primary diagnosis, with a secondary diagnosis of possible lymphoma. I had read enough Dickens to have learned about scrofula, which is due to tuberculosis spreading into the cervical lymph nodes. These are tubercular abscesses, which will sometimes open and drain, causing open wounds on the neck which continue to drain infectious discharges from the area. The senior resident gave me an amused look when he read my diagnosis. He still assumed that we would be taking a biopsy of a cancerous lymph node, but agreed that tuberculosis was reasonable to consider. I scrubbed in on her surgery and was there when he cut into the lymph node. He gave me a more respectful look over his mask and said,

"Well this does look cheesy, doesn't it?" That is exactly what a tubercular abscess looks like. On one of my earlier rotations, I had scrubbed in on surgeries of tuberculosis patients, so I was all too familiar with this disease. It helped me come to an accurate diagnosis in this case.

Naturally I was the one who took the bad news to this patient once she was back on the ward. She was relieved that it wasn't lymphoma. Even though her treatment would be no picnic, I was also able to tell her that there were medicines that would soon be available, that appeared to cure the tuberculosis, and that she may not have to stay in the sanitarium for that long a time. She was also relieved to hear that.

The ER (emergency room) was my next to last rotation and it was a very challenging experience. I saw a lot of acute trauma, major and minor, got to do some minor surgery repairing lacerations and also saw some acutely ill patients with kidney stones, heart attacks and acute infections. I was on call every third night and those were usually very busy nights. I learned a lot about making quick decisions regarding treatments and/or admission to the hospital for additional treatments or surgery. I learned about the kinds of simple triage that had to be done on very busy times when everyone seemed to be coming in at once.

On one occasion we had a young man with a severe head injury, which he sustained while taking down small trees and underbrush with a large bulldozer. One of the small trees that he was trying to uproot sprang back when he stopped the machine to take a short break. When the pressure was released the tree came back at him full force, hitting him in the head and causing several skull fractures. He was fighting the medics who were bringing him to the hospital and he continued to fight the ER staff as we tried to get an accurate assessment of the extent of his injuries. He was not conscious of what he was doing and made no responses to verbal questions or instructions. He was being prepped for immediate surgery, but blood work and skull X-rays were ordered so the surgeon would have some knowledge of the extent of his injuries. Blood and brain tissue could be seen just inside his right ear, which is something I had heard about, but never seen before. It is a very bad sign in terms of the type of fractures that can lead to that and this man's chances of survival were not good. If he survived, he would be unlikely to recover a lot of his cognitive skills and he would also likely suffer with serious sensory and/or motor deficits, meaning he might have some paralysis of his muscles and possible numbness over parts of his body.

We had gotten a portable X-ray machine and five or six of us, including some of the medics who brought him in, were trying to hold him down while one of the techs was trying to position his head long enough to get several X-rays of his head and face from multiple angles. He was a big man and very strong. I was trying to hold his left arm down while others had his other limbs and his torso as immobilized as possible. There were three other staff members standing to the side to provide additional help if needed. He suddenly put all his strength into freeing his left arm and pulled it loose. I went to catch the arm again and I suddenly realized that he was taking a swing at me. I jumped back far enough that he did not connect with me and I was then able to grab the arm and hold it down again with the help of another nurse who stepped in to help me. I apologized for losing my grip on him and she told me that my instinct to jump back at that moment probably saved me from serious injury. She said, "I thought he was going to put you through the wall." It took 10 to 15 minutes to get the X-rays taken, with enough visualization of the injuries to provide a general assessment of the injuries. As soon as that was done, he was immediately on his way to the operating room (OR). I heard later that he was still alive after the surgery, but he was on life support and not expected to live. None of us who had been restraining him had radiation protection. And someone later joked that we had just gotten our year's worth of radiation in that event.

Another patient was a traditional east Indian woman from a very conservative family. Her husband was with her and he translated for her at times. She was having severe lower abdominal pain, which had started earlier in the day. I did the history and physical exam, except I did not do a pelvic exam, thinking this needed to be done by one of the gynecology residents. I specifically asked her about whether anyone in the family had had similar symptoms and both she and her husband denied that anyone else had been ill. She had two children, but one of the other causes of this type of pain would have been an ectopic pregnancy, which seemed unlikely with her history of two normal pregnancies. The symptoms were most characteristic of pelvic inflammatory disease which would be secondary to one of the sexually transmitted infections. The gynecology resident did the pelvic exam and told us afterward that that was the most likely cause of the symptoms. We were all worried about what would happen to her and to her marriage if that is what it turned out to be. It was decided to admit her for further evaluation and to involve one of the attending physicians in the morning to help with the decision as to how to tell them what she had. By the time they started morning rounds and came to her bed, she had the classic swelling of her cheeks and lower face that is seen in mumps. The senior resident apparently asked her if her children had had mumps recently and she said immediately that her son had had mumps two weeks ago. She didn't think that was what we were talking about when we asked her if anyone in the family had been ill recently. She was kept in the hospital for about a week, as she had a fairly severe case of the mumps. She and her husband were very grateful for the good care that she had received. We were just grateful that no one had tried to talk with them the night she came in about the possibility that she had pelvic inflammatory disease. I had been unaware that mumps could present initially with inflammation of the ovaries or testicles. We had always been told that if you were too active with the mumps, or didn't rest enough, that they could "fall" on you, causing bad pain in the sexual organs.

I was in an additional quandary with this particular patient. I had personally never had a clinical case of the mumps and I had been in very close contact with her when I was examining her. She was sitting up on the exam table while I checked her eyes, nose, throat and ears. I felt her neck, looking for swelling of the lymph nodes. All this time I was also talking to her about her medical history. She would have been at her most contagious at the time I was examining her. So I made a mental note of when I would come down with the mumps and it would have been in the last month of my internship. But there was nothing much I could do about it, except wait out the verdict. I had been exposed to mumps on three different occasions as a child. Each of those times, one of my younger siblings had the mumps. I had close contact with all of them when they were sick and yet I never caught it. So I was hoping that I already had immunity to the mumps and that was confirmed when I did not become sick in the aftermath of examining that patient.

The last patient that I will discuss was a young woman who was brought into the ER, having just been in what looked initially like a minor motor vehicle accident. She had been driving in town, going about 35 mph when she collided with another car that was also driving within the speed limit. The patient did not have her seat belt on and was thrown from her car. She initially got up and looked as if she was just bruised. However, within a minute or two she began to complain of feeling weak and dizzy and she was also feeling short of breath. The policeman who had come to write up the accident said that she was starting to look like she had serious internal injuries, and he brought her in in his squad car, rather than wait for an ambulance. She was immediately placed on a gurney and I checked her pupils and her level of consciousness. Her pupils were fixed and dilated. I didn't know that was possible in someone who was still conscious enough to talk with me. She gave me her name fairly easily. She gave me only part of her address and then became less responsive. The senior resident came in at that point. The nurse had already gotten a blood pressure, which was quite low, 40/0. She was trying to get an IV started, but could not find a vein. The resident examined her chest and could not find any breathing sounds in the lower lobes of the lungs. She was struggling to breathe by then. He said that she had a hemopneumothorax, bleeding into the chest that was causing a collapsed lung. He immediately called for a chest tube set-up and stuck the chest tube in without any prep or anesthesia. She was unconscious by then. As soon as the chest tube went in, we got back bright red arterial blood and it was under pressure. Within another 30 seconds she went into cardiac arrest. I thought he would call a code and I was ready to do CPR. He shook his head and said that there was no point. She had ruptured one of the large blood vessels coming off the aorta, or possibly the aorta itself and there was nothing that could be done to save her. She had already lost most of her blood volume within the chest cavity and there was not enough time to get her to surgery, get her transfused and stop the bleeding into her chest cavity. He called for the coroner to come and he went ahead and pronounced her dead. The coroner took responsibility for notifying her mother of her death and made sure that she was sitting down before he told her that her daughter was dead.

The ER was a challenging rotation and I learned a lot while I was there. I also learned a lot by just sitting around talking with the nurses and the other house staff when things were more quiet. All of us drank coffee non-stop and most smoked cigarettes as well. To my chagrin, I developed the habit during that time even though I knew it was a bad idea. However, after one of the really rough cases, there was nothing else that leveled out my anxiety as quickly and smoothly as having a cigarette. It took me two years (four to five years later) to finally break myself of the habit. I was starting to have a chronic cough and would sometimes cough enough that I would end up gagging until I vomited. This was scary because I knew that I would have chronic lung disease very soon if I didn't stop smoking. If it hadn't been for the health issues, I doubt that I would have ever stopped smoking. I was later told by one of my teachers that nicotine is second only to cocaine in its ability to suppress intense feelings. This may be one of the reasons there are still a lot of smokers in Twelve Step groups. It is a habit that is extremely hard to break.

My last rotation was on male surgery where the rooms outside the main ward were set up as a burn unit, with two four-bed units, one male and one female. There was a two-bed room that was usually used for children. And there were also two private rooms that were usually used for the more severely burned patients. This was one of the most challenging and fascinating medical situations in which I'd been involved. If this had been my first rotation instead of my last, I would have been very tempted to become a burn surgeon.

Again, the nurses on this unit were topnotch and dealt exceptionally well with the variety of patients we had. Dealing with severely burned patients can be challenging. Many of them come in somewhat delirious due to the severe electrolyte imbalances, a result of losing so much serum from the burn sites. It would take usually up to 24 to 36 hours to stabilize one of these patients. And there were times when it would be clear to us that the patient would not survive. The nurses were very good with the patients and the family members in those situations. It made our jobs somewhat easier with their support.

The house staff consisted of myself, the first year resident and the senior resident. The first year resident was a very narcissistic man who felt entitled to work the hours he chose. He had apparently been warned about these behaviors prior to his assignment to this ward. Ten days into the rotation, he was on call and he refused to attend to a man who had not been able to urinate since his surgery, which had been done about 12 hours prior to the time he was called. As it happened, the man who was post-op and unable to void, was a good friend of the head of the department of surgery. That was the last straw for this resident and he was dismissed from the program, slightly less than three weeks before completion of his first year of residency.

That left me as the first assistant to the senior resident on all surgeries of the indigent patients. The senior resident, whose name I remember as Silas, was from one of the Amish communities in Iowa and he was a very mild-mannered man. He was very easy to work with. We made a good team and he let me do some of the closing suturing on a number of the patients. I was even able to do two appendectomies under his close supervision. I enjoyed everything about surgery except for having to get up for rounds at 6:30 a.m. Silas was somewhat amused by that and I am sure he had been getting up early most of his life. I would come in with a cup of coffee in my hand and would usually be on my second or third cup after the first case. I never saw him get upset or frustrated and he was generally soft-spoken and calm, even under very stressful circumstances. I never heard him use bad language, even at those times. He was always respectful with the patients and he seemed to be able to get the best out of anyone he was working with. It was too bad that the first year resident did not emulate him. He had been somewhat difficult to work with all along, but Silas was respectful of him in spite of his irritability and sense of entitlement. As I understood it, he was going to return to his community and provide surgical services to them in a small rural hospital. He taught me a lot during that month and I have always remembered his kindness.

I was impressed with the protocol for the treatment of the burn patients. Once they were stabilized, they would have bandages on the burned areas and the bandages were soaked in a sodium nitrate solution to promote healing of the burned areas. They were not treated prophylactally with antibiotics. Instead they had wound cultures of the burned areas once a week. If they developed a fever, indicating an infection, they would be cultured immediately and then started on an antibiotic appropriate for the organism in the most recent culture. The antibiotic would be changed only if the new culture showed a different organism. Pain medications were used as needed, and this was generally done before the daily change of dressings. Many of them did not require much pain medicine after the first 7 to 10 days.

One of the most tragic cases we had was sent from one of the rural areas. A four year old boy had been playing around the area where his parents were burning some trash. He got too close to the fire and his jeans caught on fire. His mother tried to grab him, but he was too fast. He was running as fast as he could, trying to get away from the fire, and his mother could not catch until most of his clothing was on fire. She did manage to tackle him to the ground and she used her body to smother the flames. They were brought to the hospital by the ambulance crew and the ER was ready to receive them and start their treatment. The boy was severely burned over 80 to 90% of his body, and it did not appear that he would be able to survive. He was stabilized in the ER and admitted to the four-bed male unit, as this was the only bed available. He was in pain and calling for his mother and very frightened by being in the hospital.

She was across the hall in the four-bed female room. She had burns over 40% of her body, mostly on her upper body, arms and lower face. She was in pain, but in more distress over not being able to be with her son, than she was about her own injuries. Silas spent some time with her, once both were stable medically, and let her know as gently as he could that her son was not likely to survive. He told her he would keep him as comfortable as possible and also told her he was going to keep him somewhat sedated so he would not be so stressed. Silas consulted with one of the pediatric residents about the boy's pain management and sedation and the child was sleeping most of the time after that. The nurses were very good about giving his mother reports on his condition. I believe they did help her into his room on two or three occasions so she could have some time with him.

He died late on the second day of his hospitalization. His mother was grief-stricken. The other women in her room had been very sympathetic to her from the time she arrived, and were very supportive of her once her son had died. I believe the nurses arranged for a chaplain to talk to her for a while after her son had died. She was not going to be able to attend her son's funeral as she would need to be in the hospital for several more weeks for the treatment of her burns. It was very painful for all the staff and patients in the burn unit to watch her suffering as her son lay dying in the room across the hall.

Everyone who was close to her tried to comfort her by telling her she had done everything she could to catch him and smother the flames. But she still blamed herself for not catching him as he started to run and/ or kept him further away from the fire to start with. He had been a very active child, and very impulsive, and she had just not been prepared for him to come that close to the fire that quickly. He had been warned repeatedly to stay away from the fires. But it appeared that she would have a very hard time living with her inability to get to him quickly enough to prevent him from being burned as badly as he was. She was still on the unit, and appeared very depressed, when I finished my rotation there. The nurses and her roommates continued to provide a lot of support for her and I think the chaplain remained involved as well. But I knew that she would likely carry her sadness with her for the rest of her life.

There was a young man in his late teens — I will call him Billy — who was brought in with severe electrical burns that resulted from an accident at his work. He was working on a construction crew that was putting up a silo. They were raising the center pole, to get that in place before starting the rest of the construction. A crane was being used to hoist the pole into position while Billy and three other men held chains attached to the pole, guiding it into the correct position as it was raised by the crane. Each man was placed at one of four corners to cover all the necessary angles. It was a routine procedure, until the operator of the crane hit a high-tension wire that carried a large electrical charge. Billy was standing with his left foot in a small puddle and became the transmitter for the electrical charge as it went to ground. No one else was injured, including the operator of the crane. Billy was brought to the hospital and initially stabilized in the ER. His left arm, which had been holding the chain, was essentially cooked through. He had exit burns down his back, the backs of his legs and his feet. It was not possible to tell initially how much of his left arm could be saved. He was placed in a private room because of the severity of his injuries. He was given IVs to keep his electrolytes within normal range. The burns on his back, legs and feet seemed to be a combination of second and third degree burns and he was likely going to need skin grafts on some of those burns. The most severe injury was to his left arm and it was several days before there was a clear demarcation of the healthy part of his arm and the part of his arm that was basically dead tissue that would have to be amputated.

As the demarcation became established, it was clear that he was going to lose the whole arm, with the amputation needing to be done at the shoulder. He was trying to be brave once he was stabilized, but he was clearly shaken to learn the extent of the necessary amputation. He was a football player and apparently very good at the game. The job was a summer job for him, to earn money for college. Now his football days were over, and he might even have had a football scholarship. His father was very supportive of him and spent a lot of time with him, trying to keep his spirits up. His mother was very upset and could not bear being in the room with him for very long. She could not stand to see his injury and she spent most of her time standing just outside his room. She appeared severely depressed. The nurses tried to encourage her to accept the situation for her son's sake, and I think his father tried as well. She was clearly in trouble with her own inability to accept what had happened to her son. I don't know if anyone was able to help her come to some kind of acceptance of the situation.

After seven or eight days it was time to proceed with the amputation and Billy was accepting of what was going to happen. He came back to his room post-op and had a tight bandage around the shoulder to keep pressure on the site of the amputation. He was groggy at first from the anesthesia and the pain medications, but this cleared fairly rapidly. He had become somewhat adapted to not being able to use the arm. Now he was having to adapt to not having the arm there at all. He was doing fairly well at this time and continued to try to make the most of his bad situation. His father continued to be very supportive. I rarely saw his mother. When I did she was usually out in the hall outside his room. The nurses were very good with him and he would kid around some with the ones he knew best.

I was on call and Silas and I were going over charts in the chart room when we were called to Billy's room because he was bleeding profusely from the amputation site. The nurse had been in the room with him and called for help immediately. She was applying as much pressure to the site of the bleeding as she could. She was not strong enough to completely stop the flow of blood, which was bright red arterial blood. Silas stepped in to apply more pressure and he was able to stop the bleeding. He instructed the nurse to alert the on call staff for surgery and to get everything ready to take him to the OR as fast as possible. He then turned to Billy and told him that he was going to have to take him back to surgery to tie off the artery that was bleeding. He said to him, "Before we take you to the OR I am going to have to go into the amputation site and clamp off the artery that just broke. This is going to hurt a lot, as I will have to dig into the area to find and pull out the artery so I can get the clamp on it. I don't mind if you need to curse or swear, yell or whatever you need to do, if that will make it any easier. Just don't move because I will have a harder time getting the artery if you move. Do you understand?" Billy was clearly scared but brave.

He nodded his head and said, "I won't move." The nurses had brought in one of the procedure kits that had the appropriate clamps. We both slipped on a pair of surgical gloves. Silas nodded towards the clamp he wanted and I passed it over him. He took the clamp and then dropped the bandages he had been using to keep pressure on the wound. The artery immediately began to pump out more red arterial blood. He quickly probed the wound to get hold of the artery. Billy started to curse and yell with the pain. He would have made a sailor proud. I even learned a couple of new phrases that I was unfamiliar with. But he did not move his shoulder and Silas was able to pull the artery out far enough to get the clamp on securely. He then put some bandages loosely around the clamp to stabilize it and hold it in the wound. The nurse took over keeping light pressure on the bandages and clamp to stabilize it while he was transferred to a gurney for transport to the OR. We got him to the OR in record time. A vascular surgeon had been called in to tie off the artery with Silas assisting him. I went back to the unit to work on some of the orders we had on other patients on the ward and got us caught up on that.

Billy came through the surgery without any additional problems. Silas was back after about 75 minutes and reported that he was doing well in recovery. They had ordered a hemoglobin and hematocrit post-op to get a read on how much blood he had lost. He had been typed and cross-matched for transfusions at the time of his admission and had blood waiting if he needed it. The results of the blood tests came in while we were finishing up with the charts. Silas looked at the results, which were borderline. We saw him on the unit when he returned from the recovery room and he was drowsy, but otherwise okay. He was on IV fluids to help maintain his blood volume and to provide venous access should he require a transfusion. His blood pressure was good and remaining stable. His other vitals were also stable. Silas decided to wait to see how he did overnight. If he did not have any significant changes in his blood pressure overnight he would probably not need a transfusion. He did well overnight and did not have to have a transfusion. Transfusions were not that risky in the mid-sixties, but were still not used unless necessary. Billy was young and his body appeared quite good at healing from his severe injuries. His burns were healing nicely and so far there was no evidence of infection in any of the wounds. It just did not seem necessary to transfuse him, since he would have only needed one transfusion to get him close to normal range again.

Billy was still going to be hospitalized for several weeks, possibly months, before he would be ready for discharge. I was finishing my internship a few days after his emergency surgery and I talked with him about the progress he was making, the courage he was showing and his ability to keep a positive attitude in the face of his severe injuries. He was right-handed so he would be using his dominant hand to do the work of both hands. This was much better than if he had lost his dominant hand. He talked about how much he was going to miss playing football. But he got a small grin then and said that it probably meant he would focus more on his grades and that that would be better for him in the long run. I wished him well as I was taking leave of the ward.

I told Silas how much I had enjoyed working with him and how much I had learned from him during the month. I told him that I might have been a surgeon if this had been my first rotation. He told me that I would have made a good surgeon. And then he added, "You are going to make a good psychiatrist and I think that is how this should have turned out." I also talked with the nurses and told them how much I had enjoyed working with them on the unit. They were a special group of nurses and did an excellent job of watching the ward patients and also closely monitoring the small burn unit. I also told them that I felt like I was a competent physician for the more common medical problems patients have, and that I owed that knowledge to the rotating internship that I had completed there. It was hard to leave the hospital, my fellow interns and the challenges that I had learned to deal with over the course of the year.

I packed my things and left early on June 30, 1967 for the trip back to Charlottesville and my residency at the University of Virginia Hospital.

CHAPTER SEVEN

Residency: The First Three Years

When I started my residency I was glad to be back, as I had a number of friends there who were classmates in medical school. But I was amazed by the transformation of the university, and to a lesser extent, of the medical school. When I left just one year earlier, the school was a very traditional, coat and tie school. All the men were clean-shaven. The undergraduates were all men and the undergraduate women were from Sweetbriar or one of the other all female universities. The graduate schools and the medical school had a few women, but the vast majority of the students were male. When I returned to the University in 1967, there were still some men who continued the traditional look, but a lot of the students were much more casually dressed, and there were a lot of beards and mustaches. There were also a lot of hippies and there was a significant drug scene; marijuana was readily available. The other drug that was very popular was LSD. There were a number of younger teenagers, many of whom were runaways. I do not recall a lot of organized protests, but the climate seemed similar to Berkley, where some of the major protests took place. It was a time of major transition for the nation and these were the youths that epitomized the coming changes.

As a first year resident I was assigned to the inpatient service for the year. We had eight residents, so I was on call every eighth night. This felt almost like a luxury, but we still worked very hard on the nights we were on call. During the first seven or eight months, we had frequent calls to the ER to admit acutely psychotic young men or, less frequently, women, who were having their first experience with LSD, and were having very bad trips. They would usually be admitted to the psychiatric unit for a few days. Most of their symptoms cleared quickly with fairly low doses of Thorazine or Mellaril, and they would be discharged within three or four days. Most did not require any follow-up. A few would not clear and in most instances these turned out to be young men with their first episode of schizophrenia, precipitated by the LSD, but most would likely have had a psychotic break at some point anyway. By the end of the first year, we were no longer seeing the acute, drug-related episodes, but were seeing instead the individuals who remained psychotic after several days. The students, who were experimenting with these drugs, mainly LSD and marijuana, had learned how to stop a bad trip the same way we did on the unit, with low to moderate doses of Thorazine and Mellaril. They had been able to find supplies of these medications and were managing the bad trips on their own.

During my first year of medical school, a student had been arrested and convicted of possession of marijuana, and he was sentenced to 20 years in prison for the offense. By the time I returned for my residency, there were changes in the penalties for possession, with much less severe consequences for minor drug-related offenses. There were also individuals who were beginning to push for the legalization of marijuana. It is only in recent years that we have been able to begin serious decriminalization of that drug. The war on drugs has been going on for thirty to forty years, and has been an utter failure as far as making street drugs unavailable to the average citizen. Marijuana is now legal for recreational use in several states, and is now legal for medical use in over half the states in the nation. The states that have taken this step are now running budget surpluses from the taxes they collect on the marijuana, which is taxed in the same way that cigarettes and alcohol are taxed. But the initial widespread use of marijuana had become an integral part of the social scene within the one brief year I was in Iowa.

The psychiatric inpatient units were on the second and third floor of one of the older buildings of the original hospital. They were in the Davis wing, and were designated as Davis 2 for the second floor unit, and Davis 3 for the third floor unit. This wing was also connected to the Barringer wing, which housed neurology and other services. Both wings were connected to the new hospital, which was a six-floor building with all the latest technology for patient care readily available in every patient room. Many of the rooms were semi-private and the rest were private. The medical, surgical, pediatric, obstetrics and gynecology services were all in the new hospital. Psychiatry and neurology shared the space in the older building.

Each psychiatric inpatient unit had at least one four-bed room and the rest were semi-private and private rooms. To give you an idea of the standard costs of psychiatric inpatient care, the daily cost of the four-bed room was \$40/patient, the cost of the semi-private room was \$42/patient and the cost of the private room was \$44/patient. I have no idea why I remember those prices, but I do. The nurses station/charting area was to the left when you entered the unit. Next on the left were two seclusion rooms, where patients were placed when they were severely agitated or presented an immediate risk to themselves and/or to others. There was an office located between the seclusion rooms on one of the floors, and the on-call room, where the on-call resident slept was between the seclusion rooms on the other floor. Across the hall from the nurses station/charting area was another smaller office space where the nurses gave report and it was also used for talking with patients privately at times or taking a smoke break when necessary. When I was on call I would sit in on the nurses report if I could, to know what the patients' overall conditions were. I would frequently take a smoke break with one or more of the nurses, which gave us a chance to talk about patients, or to just unwind by shooting the breeze on one of the slower nights.

All of the residents had office space assigned where we could see inpatients and, occasionally outpatients, who were frequently patients that we had taken care of during their inpatient hospitalization. Some of the patients that I saw in this way, I saw for the four years that I was a resident there. We were encouraged to work with the patients in on-going, psychoanalytically oriented psychotherapy and we got excellent supervision for the psychotherapy that we did. Several of the attending staff were fully trained psychoanalysts and several others were doing their psychoanalytic training at the Washington Psychoanalytic Institute in Washington, D.C.

The Diagnostic and Statistical Manual, which was used to make diagnostic assessments of our patients, was in its second revision and it was psychoanalytic in its orientation. It was called DSM-2 for short. Shortly after I finished my residency, the DSM-3 came out and it completely did away with the psychoanalytic orientation. It was set up to be symptom based and was structured to try to make the diagnoses more reproducible over the lifetime of the patient. With DSM-2, diagnoses frequently changed from one hospitalization or treatment course to a later one. With the advent of medications that effectively treated depression, anxiety and psychotic disorders, there was a need by the pharmaceutical companies for homogenous groups, all sharing roughly the same set of symptoms, so that more effective clinical trials of new medications would be possible. This way of diagnosing took away the life experience of individual patients, which, would, many times, give continuity to the history of their illness, in favor of using symptoms as the primary diagnostic criteria. Structured diagnostic interviews became a standard for assessing individual patients. There are now a multitude of standardized tests that are used for diagnosis. Also statistics has become a primary influence in the assessment and treatment of patients. Some of the non-medication treatments, especially cognitive behavioral therapies, have standardized manuals that are used by the therapist and the patient in the treatment process. As some of these treatments have become acceptable to insurance reviewers, because they are considered best practices or are evidenced-based, they are much easier to get reimbursement for than psychoanalytically oriented therapies. The DSM was just revised again (there have been several revisions of both 3 and 4) and in May of 2014 the American Psychiatric Association came out with DSM-5, which has a much larger number of diagnoses than any of the previous revisions. And they have eliminated Asperger's Disorder, one of the autistic spectrum disorders, from the manual for reasons that are not entirely clear to me. It was always a useful diagnosis as it was an autistic disorder without significant speech delays. I have always considered that a significant distinction.

At this point I have taken a bit of a detour in my account of my first year of residency. I found the DSM-2 very useful for understanding and diagnosing my patients. I was still doing the diagnostic formulation at the end of my admission history and physical. I still believe that this was the best way to summarize the individual's illness and its determinants. I continue to use this method of understanding my patients to this day and still find it extremely helpful. I have had direct experience with treating people in psychoanalysis and, also from my own personal analysis, and it is a very powerful tool for helping someone to heal from the early traumas of their lives. There are still practicing psychoanalysts in large cities but that treatment is generally for people who can pay for the treatment out of pocket, without insurance reimbursement. But during my residency this treatment was available to a lot of middle class patients through the major medical part of their insurance coverage. All the federal insurances covered it this way with a $50,000 limit on that coverage. The $50,000 could be used for any lengthy physical or mental illness and this was a life-time limit for all such illnesses. The fees for psychoanalytic therapies were $30 to $40 per session and quite a few federal employees got a full analysis with their major medical coverage. The federal plans also covered 365 days of inpatient treatment, which allowed long term treatment in hospitals like McLean in Boston, Shepherd-Pratt in Baltimore and Chestnut Lodge in Rockville, MD, just outside of D.C. Chestnut Lodge is the hospital in the book *I Never Promised You a Rose Garden*. There were other hospitals in other large cities around the nation that provided this kind of long-term treatment. All of them are now closed except for Shepherd-Pratt and McLean. These treatments have now become available only to the wealthier individuals who can pay out of pocket for their care.

Well, that was my second detour. Now back to my first year of residency. Each resident was assigned to six months on one of the units and then did the second six months on the other unit. There were different attendings on each unit and the attending for that unit was my primary supervisor for that six months. Both were in psychoanalytic training and that was the focus of therapy during that year.

One of the unexpected results of the medications for treatment of tuberculosis, was the observation that patients on one of these particular medications seemed to get better with their depression as well as their tuberculosis. This led to the development of the first class of anti-depressants, called MAO inhibitors, which were effective for depression, but had serious side effects of elevated blood pressure if the patient ate aged cheeses or drank red wines and there were several other foods that could also cause that problem. This first group of anti-depressants was shortly followed by the tricyclic anti-depressants, Tofranil and Elavil, both of which were very effective and lacked the side effects of the MAO inhibitors. Anti-anxiety drugs were readily available with Librium and Valium being the main ones during the early part of my residency. I have already mentioned the anti-psychotic medications, Thorazine and Mellaril, which were effective for our bipolar and schizophrenic patients. Stelazine and Trilafon, additional anti-psychotic medications, were also available shortly thereafter.

Medication usage was becoming another tool for the treatment of mental illness and was challenging both the psychotherapies and electro-convulsive therapy (ECT) as more effective treatments that worked faster than therapy and had less side effects than ECT. I did some ECT as part of my training, and I have at times referred patients with treatment-resistant depression for ECT to get improvement in the depression when medication alone has not been effective. But except for the time in my residency, I have not done ECT in any of my practices. But I have always utilized medications along with therapy for most of my patients except during the time I was in psychoanalytic training and in a psychoanalytic therapy practice in D.C., when I did primarily therapy without the use of medication. Since leaving that practice I have used mostly medications with supportive therapy with a few psychoanalytic therapy patients also as part of my practice. I learned to use the combinations of treatments during my residency and still feel I got excellent training in both approaches during that time.

During my second year of residency I had six months on the consultation-liason service, doing psychiatric evaluations on medically ill patients who were on the regular medical and surgical units. The second six months was at the mental health center, which was housed across the street from the hospital, and was exclusively outpatient evaluations and treatments. This was in the era of the downsizing of the large, state mental hospitals, which up until then, had treated the chronically mentally ill with long-term admissions, many of them life-long. Schizophrenic patients typically did not leave the state hospital. Bipolar disorder, then called manic-depressive illness, was considered a better prognosis illness, as many of them could be discharged after three to five years, with good improvement in their mood symptoms.

There was an unfortunate political trend at the time, that blamed a lot of the patients' symptoms on the institutions where they were hospitalized, and there were multiple groups advocating for the closure of the long term hospitals, describing them as coercive and dehumanizing institutions, which were harmful to patients instead of helpful. This also came to include places like the Lynchburg Colony, which was seen as detrimental to the lives of severely retarded individuals, as well as severely physically disabled children. With each of these long-term institutions, my experience was that they generally provided good care for severely disabled adults and children, under very difficult circumstances. Many of the people, who were the caregivers to these patients, were the third or fourth generation in their families to have provided such care in these institutions. These were families committed to the care of these patients over several generations and they were personally invested in providing the best care they could for these unfortunates.

Most of the Virginia state hospitals have become short-term hospitals, and they only keep patients a few weeks longer than the private hospitals. Most of these people are not faring well outside the old wards. Many of them have become criminalized and are living in a truly coercive and dehumanizing institution, namely state, private and a small number of federal penal institutions. They do get some treatment in the prison setting, but once they are released, they frequently become homeless and vulnerable to people who prey on them and exploit them. Others are in group homes, which are limited, and some in subsidized and supervised housing. Others remain with their families, and the families frequently suffer significant problems trying to care for these patients, who can consume a large part of the family's resources due to their special needs.

There was one tragic patient, a middle-aged man who had spent most of his adult life in one of the state institutions. He was diagnosed with schizophrenia and when he was discharged from the hospital, he was assigned a case manager to monitor his outpatient services, and sent home to his mother, who was elderly and not in good health. He had had numerous visits to the ER for complaints of suicidal ideation and voices commanding him to kill himself. He was on medication, but remained unstable. He had had two or three re-hospitalizations back at the state hospital, but would always be discharged within two or three months. When I started at the clinic, I was told about this man's constant attempts to get back into the hospital. These attempts were to be handled differently from now on. He was to be seen more often by his case worker and he would be seen on an emergency basis at the mental health center, but would just be given more intensive outpatient services and not re-hospitalized again.

I did not see him as a patient. But I will not forget the day that one of the staff spotted him trudging up the walkway to the clinic, at the top of the hill. Several of the staff gathered around the window to watch his progress. He had been told at a prior appointment that he would not be sent back to the hospital again. I was also watching him from my window and I saw him stop just before he reached the entrance to the clinic. He stood there, staring at the clinic entrance, with a hopeless look on his face. He stood there for several minutes and then started to shake his head in a negative way. He then turned around and started walking back down the walkway, back toward his home. Several staff were delighted and believed that he would now commit to the outpatient treatment that had been set up for him. But he did not. He went home that afternoon and killed himself. He could not adjust to life outside the hospital and it cost him his life.

Frannie

During my first year of residency, a woman, whom I shall call Frannie (short for Frances), was admitted to Davis II. She was around 30 years old and was admitted for treatment of her depression and suicidal impulses. She was not my patient, but I remember her very well, because of her history. She had been admitted to one of the long-term, state hospitals with severe, chronic and treatment-resistant depression. She had been psychotic at times, with paranoid delusions and auditory hallucinations. It was thought for some time that she had some form of schizophrenia and was not expected to leave the hospital. For a period of about 10 months she had been in a catatonic state, lying motionless in bed, with a feeding tube for nourishment and a Foley catheter for urine output. She was given excellent care, and required total care of all her basic needs during that time. After about 10 months she began to slowly come out of the catatonic state. She began to help with some of her care and she started to have some communication with the hospital staff who took care of her. Within a month she began to walk again, though she needed assistance with walking for the first several weeks. She had been completely bedfast for 10 months and had to relearn to walk and become independent in her self care. It took her some time to regain the strength in her muscles to be able to do all these things.

She became more active on the unit and began to go out on the grounds of the hospital, taking short walks with some of the other patients. She improved gradually over the next several months and was interacting with both staff and other patients. She continued to improve and began to talk about leaving the hospital. I do not know what had happened to her parents. She made contact with an aunt and uncle, who began to visit her in the hospital. They were willing to have her live with them when she left the hospital. She started having weekend passes with them and the visits went well. She then went on passes that lasted for 7 to 10 days and eventually she was allowed a 30 day pass. At the end of that pass she felt ready to leave the hospital, and she was discharged.

At the time she came into Davis II she had been out of the hospital for almost a year and had been functioning reasonably well during the first six to eight months. She then began to have more depression, with problems with sleep and appetite. She was beginning to feel more anxious and was easily overwhelmed. She began to feel hopeless about her life and started to think about suicide. Her aunt and uncle became worried about her and had her admitted to the University Hospital. She did not want to go back to the state hospital because she would be a failure and never able to leave again. She was being seen at one of the mental health centers in the area where she lived with her aunt and uncle. She was also on medications for depression and psychosis. She was somewhat overwhelmed when she was first admitted to the unit. She tended to stay to herself and did not interact much with staff or with the other patients. She was usually up most of the night and she would talk with the night nurses some as she got more used to the unit. She needed a lot of support and encouragement to take part in any of the daytime activities, but at times she would sit in on the group sessions, though she did not actively participate.

On one of the nights I was on call, I was sitting in on the shift change report at 11 p.m. The night nurse had developed a good relationship with Frannie and she asked if I would see her that night if she was willing to talk with me. I agreed to do it, since it was a slow night, and I was caught up on everything. The nurse had seen Frannie pacing up and down the hall, as she came on the unit, and could tell that she was more agitated than usual. I stayed in the small room, where the nurses were doing report, and she brought Frannie to me after report was over.

She was very shy at first and did not make eye contact. She sat quietly for a few minutes and I let her know that I was there to hear about what was bothering her that night. I didn't say anything else and simply waited for her to begin to talk. After several minutes she began to talk about being in the state hospital and the very conflicted feelings she was having about her experience there. She had felt better being with her aunt and uncle and did not know why she got depressed again. She was afraid that she was a hopeless case. She did not feel that she could talk in group because she was afraid that no one would believe her. She was also afraid of offending some of the other patients, but could not be specific about what she thought would be offensive. She talked about not knowing what to do with her life, as she felt she needed to help her aunt and uncle, since they had been kind enough to take her in. She also felt that she was different from the other patients, because she had been in the state hospital, and it made her uncomfortable to think about the other patients knowing that about her. I asked if she listened to the other patients' concerns when they were talking about their fears and she said that she did. I asked her why she thought her fears were any different from theirs, even though her life experience was different from most of theirs. She thought about that for several minutes without saying anything. Then she said she had never thought her fears would be similar to the fears that others had.

She then began to talk about being in the hospital bed for all those months, because she was too afraid to do anything but lay very still all the time. I asked if she could remember what was going on around her during that time and she said that she was very aware of everything. She just did not feel safe enough to respond to any of the things going on around her. I then asked her what had allowed her to begin to reclaim her life and begin to interact again with the staff and patients. She thought about that for several minutes and said it just seemed like the right time. She felt more secure in that situation at that point. I asked if part of her fears on the unit were similar to her fears before she went into the completely withdrawn state. She again thought about her answer for several minutes. She then acknowledged that her fears in both situations were similar. She was starting to see the fears on the unit as not that unique and, perhaps for the first time, that she was not the only one with fears that could be overwhelming. She started to relax and she made eye contact for the first time in the session. She said then that she always thought that she was completely alone with the fears, and that no one would understand. She admitted that she had had other patients at the state hospital voice similar fears and that that had helped her feel less afraid in the hospital. I talked about the fears being something that everyone has to deal with at some time in their lives, and the hospital unit being a safe place to learn about one's own unique version of the fears and anxieties. She was thoughtful for a few minutes and I then asked her why she had taken the profound withdrawal from everything for all those months, as what seemed to her the safest way to deal with her fears. She looked at me for several minutes without answering. Then she said, "I just needed the time." She then talked about being cared for all that time, like a young child, and finally realizing that she didn't have to do that any more. She did not think of leaving the hospital at the time, just that she could take part in the life on the unit and could be safe doing it. I then suggested that she was now facing a more grown-up version of those same fears, and doing it without the profound withdrawal she had needed in the state hospital. She sat quietly for several more minutes and then thanked me for talking with her. She said she felt sleepy and thought she might sleep the rest of the night for the first time in months. She then went back to her room and I went to the on-call room for the night. The night nurse told me the next time I was on call, that she had really benefitted from the talk that night, and that she was taking a more active role on the unit. I saw her in passing several more times before I went off the inpatient units as I started my second year of residency. She always made eye contact and greeted me with a smile and we always said "Hi" to each other. She was still on Davis II when I went to the consult service and I never heard anything else about what happened to her.

Carl

One of the most difficult patients I had early in my first year of residency, was a young man I shall call Carl. He was brought in through the ER, having been picked up by the police, because he was out in the middle of one of the busy highways leading into Charlottesville, with a hand full of his medicine, flagging down motorists and warning them that there were poisons in the medications. He was clearly psychotic, but was also confused at times. I was on call that night and I saw him in the emergency room and quickly admitted him to the psychiatric unit. He was admitted to a regular bed, but I immediately placed him in one of the seclusion rooms because of his high level of agitation. He was very paranoid about his medication, which the hospital pharmacy quickly identified as methotrexate, an oral medication for the treatment of cancer. I put him on one on one close observation and one of our orderlies (now he would be called a CNA or certified nursing assistant) was sitting with him, close by his hospital bed in the seclusion room. I gave him a moderate dose of Thorazine intramuscular (IM) and he began to calm down. I was then able to talk to him for about 10 or 15 minutes, learning that he was a graduate student in one of the basic sciences, that he was married and had a 4-year-old daughter. He also disclosed that he had been treated for a lymphoma about two years prior to this admission. He gave me permission to talk with his wife who was now waiting outside the unit, having been informed by the police of his whereabouts.

I met with his wife in my office and she gave me his medical history in more detail. He had had a lymphoma involving the lower spine, and had had radiation for that about two years before. They had been afraid that he would become paraplegic as he had had some numbness and weakness of his legs initially, which is what led him to seek medical treatment at the time. However, he had had an excellent response to the radiation, with complete clearing of the lymphoma tumor pressing on his spine. The numbness and weakness also cleared and he had no problems with his legs after that. He was being continued on the methotrexate to prevent any recurrence of the lymphoma. He had been free of any evidence of cancer for the past two years and had been symptom free until his sudden onset of mental status changes, which rapidly worsened over a 24-hour period, until he left the home without any explanation. His wife did not know where he had gone, but she had contacted the police to tell them he was missing and that he was having some kind of nervous breakdown. That was how they had known how to get in touch with her when they found him on the highway. He had remained agitated but manageable while he was in the police car and they stayed with him in the ER until we could get him safely onto the unit and in a safe situation in the seclusion room. His wife indicated that he had no history of prior mental illness and that he had never been paranoid or psychotic. Needless to say, she was very worried about him. She asked if this could be related to his cancer treatments and I said that was one of things I would be evaluating. I let her on the unit to see him for a few minutes, and he seemed calmer after talking with her. Clearly, they had a good relationship.

I did the admission history and physical, and in my brief neurological exam, could find no abnormalities. I was very grateful for the month of neurology that I had during my internship as I knew what to order initially. I did the usual screening labs, but also requested a neurology consult and ordered a brain scan. My differential included depression and psychosis related to the stress of dealing with a potentially terminal illness as well as the possibility of a lymphoma metastasis to the brain. My supervisor did not think the brain scan was in order and felt that the stress of his illness was the most likely cause of his symptoms. I knew that the brain scan would yield information by the end of the afternoon and would be useful information for the neurology resident when he did the consult. I got a call from radiology that afternoon that he had a large tumor in the left temporal area of his brain. They sent up a copy of the images and there was no mistaking the danger this represented for him. I notified the neurology resident of the scan results and he came to see him late in the afternoon. He had gotten the old chart of his previous treatment which had been done at the University Hospital, and had more information on the type of lymphoma and the treatment history. He requested neurosurgery to see him as they had been involved with his initial treatment. With the history of an excellent response to radiation, they made the decision that

that would likely be the most reasonable treatment to offer him. They did sedate him and take him to surgery to do a biopsy of the mass to make sure that it was the same lymphoma, which it was.

Ordinarily he would have been transferred to the neurosurgery floor, for the biopsy and follow-up treatment. However, his ongoing severe agitation and paranoia could not be safely managed on the neurosurgery unit. He could be somewhat combative at times and needed the seclusion room and the support of one on one supervision to keep the behaviors in check. The neurology resident indicated that he would likely become worse with his agitation and psychosis during the initial radiation treatments, because the brain and the tumor will normally swell in response to the radiation, putting more pressure on the brain before the tumor begins to shrink. In about 45 minutes, the three of us residents, along with the head nurse on the unit were able to put together a treatment plan that included all of his radiation, neurosurgery and neurology treatments while he continued to be a patient on the psychiatric unit. I'm not sure that that could be done in the same way now.

Wellmont-Bristol Regional Medical Center in Bristol, Tennessee had a medical-psychiatric unit, which could have provided the type of care that Carl received. It had been one of only a few of these units nationwide. It was changed to a gero-psych unit two or three years ago. These units are limited to geriatric patients, with the age limit set at 60 or older. There may be a few units that will accept people in their late fifties. On the other hand, the radiation treatments are much more focused and better tolerated now than they were in 1967, and would likely be more manageable on a surgical or medical floor.

Carl indeed had a worsening of his agitation, confusion and psychotic symptoms during the first week of treatment. He remained under control with the constant supervision and his isolation in the seclusion room. I also ordered regular doses of Thorazine 100 mg four times a day, and as needed (PRN) injections of 50 mg of Thorazine for worsening agitation or times when he threatened to become combative. The orderlies were very experienced in dealing with out of control patients and were calm and supportive, but firm with him during that first week. Early in the second week, he began to improve. The first sign of this was the decreased need for the PRN doses of the Thorazine. By the middle of the second week he was allowed to take walks up and down the hall and he began to interact with some of the other patients. I kept him in the seclusion room at night for two or three more days. By then he no longer had the paranoia or the confusion. He was not agitated and was fully aware of his situation by then. I had continued to see him briefly once or twice a day while he was completely confined to the seclusion room. I would help him stay oriented to his being in a hospital and receiving treatment for the lymphoma in his brain. He began to be able to talk with me more lucidly toward the end of the first week. During the early part of the second week, I was able to start seeing him in my office, though I limited the sessions to 20 to 30 minutes in duration, so as not to cause him undue stress. By the time I released him from the seclusion room, and he was in a regular patient bed in one of the semi-private rooms, he was taking part in all the activities on the unit. I would see him for a full session of 50 minutes three times a week and daily for a few minutes during morning rounds.

He was a very intelligent young man and had no illusions about his prognosis with the lymphoma. He experienced a lot of sadness about his illness and the knowledge that he most likely would not live to see his daughter grow up. I was supportive of his grieving during the private sessions and he was able to tell me that he had had some depression about his situation for several months before he was brought to the hospital. He had kept this from his wife as he did not want to worry her. He was open to a trial of an anti-depressant for his depression and I started him on Tofranil, working the dose up to 150 mg daily over the next 10 days. I was also able to reduce his Thorazine dose to 50 mg three times a day during the six to eight weeks that he remained in the hospital.

He completed the radiation treatments in six weeks and was to continue under the care of the oncologist that he had seen prior to his admission to the hospital. He was to continue on a different combination of anti-cancer medications and these were started following completion of his radiation treatments. I saw him in follow-up six weeks after his discharge and he reported doing well on just the Tofranil. He no longer felt depressed and he was now back in school and doing the make-up work he had missed due to his hospitalization. He elected to continue on the Tofranil through his internist and I did not expect to see him again.

He did come back to see me during the spring of my second year, while I was in the mental health center. He requested to see me so he could talk about his feelings about his worsening medical issues with the lymphoma. He was no longer taking the Tofranil and reported having good days and bad days. He was aware of sadness over his terminal condition and did not want to burden his wife with these issues. He had at most about 6 to 12 months to live according to his oncologist. He talked about trying to live each day to the fullest. He continued to enjoy his relationship with his daughter and the changes he could see as she got older. She was in a kindergarten class and enjoying being in school. He continued to have a close relationship with his wife, but he did try to be optimistic about his situation with her, because she became anxious and sad when he seemed to be having a bad day or a setback. I let him talk about these issues for most of the session. He seemed to get a lot of relief from talking about these issues. He did continue to have good days when he did not feel the depression or sadness. He worked very hard to make every day a good day, and felt he was successful most of the time. I did not suggest restarting the Tofranil as he did not appear to have significant depression. He did have appropriate sadness about his limited life expectancy. I left it open for him to return for additional appointments if he needed to. He indicated that he would and said that our talk had been helpful.

The next time I saw him was about 18 months later. He had been admitted to the neurology service with some non-specific symptoms of lethargy and occasional confusion. They consulted me (I was not on the consult service at that time) because they had done a thorough work-up without finding any significant changes in his medical status to explain his symptoms. They had requested that I see him, since I had been the primary psychiatrist involved in his care. I agreed to see him and saw him in the late afternoon after completing my work on the inpatient unit, where I was the senior resident. He was very withdrawn and it was an effort for him to say anything much to me in response to my initial questions. He was not confused. I sat for a few minutes without saying anything and he seemed to relax a little. I had watched people in the process of dying while I was an intern, and I had seen a number of them become quieter and more withdrawn within the few days before they died. They seemed to be pulling away from this world, and they appeared to be almost in preparation for leaving it. It's not that they were pulling away from their families or the staff. They seemed to want someone with them, but they were not able to talk much with whoever was there. It seemed to take most of their energy to do simple responses to questions such as, "How are you feeling?" As I sat there silently for those few minutes, I was recalling these patients, and I sadly recognized that Carl appeared to be in a similar process. I then asked if he was in pain and he shook his head for "no". I then asked if he was comfortable with me sitting with him for awhile and he nodded. I remained with him for another 20 minutes. I was thinking about the fact that I was going to be away for the next few days, to a medical conference, and I did not expect him to live long enough for me to see him again. Nevertheless, I explained to him that I would be at the conference for the next few days, and that I would be back at the end of the week. I told him that I would see him again on Friday, if he was still in the hospital. He just nodded again. I held his hand for a moment before I left and told him I would tell the neurologist that he did not need any additional medications for now. He nodded again and said "Thank you." I then left and spoke with the neurology resident, telling him that I did not think his condition was due to depression so much as it was sadness at being so close to death. He acknowledged that that was a possibility as his condition appeared to be deteriorating, in spite of the fact that they could not pinpoint any one thing in his condition that should be immediately life-threatening. I thought about Carl during the time I was at the conference. As soon as I got back, I contacted the neurology resident who informed me that he had died quietly about two days after I had last seen him. He was not able to leave the hospital before his death.

By the third year of my residency there were a number of changes sweeping the university including the Department of Psychiatry.

We had a new faculty member who was analytically trained from the Washington Psychoanalytic Institute and who was also experienced with group therapies, including the sensitivity groups that were coming into vogue in a number of situations nation-wide. He started a group within the department that included a wide variety of individuals, including a chaplain, one of the psychologists, a few medical students and some administrative staff as well as nurses, residents and other clinical staff. We were a group of about 14 or 15 individuals and we met regularly for about nine to ten months that year. We met once a week to observe our process with each other and with the group to help us better understand the ways in which the group could be dysfunctional as well as ways to move in the direction of being higher functioning. It was my first participation in an experience that facilitated understanding how to be genuinely productive in spite of interpersonal problems and it led me to undertake my personal analysis to deal with my own depression.

During the first four months of the third year I worked in the Child and Adolescent Department and was able to work with several patients and their families on a short-term basis, dealing with issues varying from attention deficit disorder to anxiety to childhood depression. We did visit the Children's Rehabilitation Center for one day of that rotation to see the range of services available to children with intellectual and/or physical deficits.

During the second four months I was split between the mental health center and a new program, the Crisis Service that was relatively new. The team consisted of a senior resident who was also based at the mental health center, an attending psychiatrist and a social worker. We were developing a model for short-term admissions, to try to do an intensive intervention with a patient in crisis. These patients were on the regular inpatient units, but the treatment team was different. One of the nurses was usually assigned to go on rounds with us in the morning, so I had a lot of contact with the nursing staff during that time The Crisis Service became a very useful service for patients who had limited or no insurance coverage for mental health services, and it was still in place at the time I finished my residency and moved on to Washington, D.C.

For the Crisis service the patient was usually admitted through the ER and a treatment plan was rapidly developed and implemented, with the mobilization of outpatient psychiatric and therapeutic services usually scheduled within the first 24 to 36 hours of the admission. Medications were started and benefits and side effects assessed daily from the time of the admission. This was part of my third year mental health center rotation as these patients usually followed up with us in the clinic following discharge. The social worker would meet with family members within the first two days and helped to develop a treatment plan that included therapy with the patient and the family, to promote good family support following the hospitalization. The maximum time for the admission was five days and, for the most part, we were able to have the patient ready for discharge within three to five days. On rare occasions when they required a longer stay, usually due to medication problems or a poor or absent support system at home, they would be transitioned to one of the regular inpatient units. The work was demanding and time-consuming, but we got very good results in many instances and I learned a lot about managing patients in the short run.

It was during the time that I was on the Crisis Service that I was able to observe the beginnings of some major changes on Davis III. This was the result of another sensitivity group, this one involving just the clinical staff of the unit meeting once weekly to process important issues on the unit. Sometimes this was focused on problems with particular patients and sometimes it focused on problems with how the staff was handling conflict between differing opinions and approaches within the clinical staff. By the time I was on the Crisis Service they had begun to talk about changing the way things were done on the unit in favor of trying to use an approach that had been developed in England. There were several ways of doing this and most often this was identified as the development of a therapeutic community. The idea behind this was that patients were active members of the ward community and could provide feedback to the staff about some of the decisions that affected them and their treatment. It was also about creating a more egalitarian atmosphere in the ward community and respecting the patients' active participation in their own therapeutic process, rather than viewing them as passive recipients of treatment plans made by people who were viewed as their superiors and experts not to be questioned. I had been observing the transition of the Davis III unit during the months leading up to the birth of the therapeutic community, from listening to the feedback of the residents who were on the unit during that time, as well as that of the nursing staff. I was also able to observe when I was there as the back up for the first year resident on call, when there were several admissions late in the day. During times that I was there in the evening as I was charting on the unit, I had the opportunity to quietly watch the effects of such dramatic changes in protocols. The therapeutic community was put into place two weeks before I was to rotate off the Crisis Service and start my final four months of that year as the senior resident on Davis III. By then I was looking forward to this new experience and very much in favor of the changes that had been put in place.

One of the important changes was the morning group meeting, which involved all the patients on the unit who were able to participate plus all the clinical staff including nurses, residents, medical students, the unit psychologist and the attending psychiatrist. Everyone was able to bring up issues they were concerned about and anyone could provide suggestions and additional observations as they saw fit. Patients' input was given the same respect and attention as that of staff members. The meetings were conducted in an informal way but disrespectful comments were confronted as a barrier to open communication. There remained rules, of course, but when it was time for a patient to come off of suicide precautions, for example, or be given permission to leave the building to walk around the grounds, it was the fellow patients — the community, if you will, that had input regarding the wisdom of the decision. It put everything out in the open. There was no "snitching" in private. The patients would be genuinely concerned when one was not being honest with the staff about what was going on, or if someone was getting worse. This responsibility for each other was also therapeutic for the patients, as it gave them more autonomy in terms of their own illnesses, by being helpful to others.

One of the issues we were facing immediately had to do with the attending psychiatrist, who was responsible for the supervision of the unit activities, as well as the direct supervisor of the individual residents' therapy sessions with the patients that they were directly responsible for. The attending on Davis III at the time the therapeutic community was started, was not a supporter of the changes on the unit. I do not know how active he had been in the staff meetings prior to my rotation in to the unit as senior resident. He was not very active in the staff meetings and he frequently missed the morning community meetings. Also word was coming down that the chairman of the Department of Psychiatry was not a fan of the changes. In spite of all that, I was a strong supporter of the community and that was enough to keep it going, particularly since there were no actual attempts to get us to go back to the previous way of organizing the unit.

I had not been present for any of the staff meetings for Davis III during the time the therapeutic community was being developed. I joined those staff meetings when I started as the senior resident on Davis III. These meetings continued for the remainder of that year. The staff was initially somewhat concerned about how I would respond to the changes in how the unit was run. I had been in a sensitivity group with the psychiatrist who was running the staff group for the unit for the previous seven or eight months and I was already familiar with some of the new concepts involved in the unit being changed into a therapeutic community. So contrary to the staff's concerns, I was very interested in continuing the plan the unit staff had put in place, and I let them know very quickly that I would continue what they had started, since it was a method of treatment that gave the patients much more autonomy with respect to decisions made regarding their treatment process. Additionally, I found the concept of a therapeutic community very exciting and began to read some of the books and literature, mostly from United Kingdom sources, that described the origins of these treatment facilities in England.

The day on the unit began after the patients had had breakfast, and was a meeting of the staff and patients that looked at the current issues and/or problems on the unit, with the discussion being focused on looking for solutions to problems, with input from both staff and patients. Some of the unit rules and procedures were modified based on patients' input in these meetings. They were usually done on a trial basis, and the success and/or difficulties with these changes continued to be monitored in the morning community meetings. Sometimes the changes were not that effective and would not be continued further. Most times the changes were of benefit to the functioning of the unit, making it truly a therapeutic experience for the patients and, also frequently, for the staff as well.

The other unit, Davis II, continued to operate in the traditional way, and this was a good unit with good therapeutic results as well. The patients on Davis II just did not have input as to policies on the unit, or input as to decisions affecting other patients' status in the community, i.e., was a specific patient ready to go on outings with the other patients or ready for a home pass for a few hours. These were decisions to which the patients on Davis III had input, when they were being discussed in the community meetings. The differences in the two units would actually give the residents and medical students a broader experience of inpatient treatments, since the two units gave two different experiences, both of which had their advantages and disadvantages. Medical students also frequently took part in the community meetings, and quickly became used to providing input on their observations of the patients and the unit, just as everyone else did. All staff gave input, from the nursing assistants right up to the senior psychiatrist, and the patients gave input as well. Everyone's contribution was respected and the unit functioned in a more egalitarian way. It was much less hierarchical than more traditional medical and psychiatric units.

David

Shortly after I became the senior resident on Davis III, we had a young man, whom I will call David, admitted to the unit with an acute and severe psychosis. The police brought him into the ER because he was making threats to harm himself and/or others. He was admitted directly to the unit and placed in the seclusion room. Initially he was severely agitated and begging for someone to stop the voices that were telling him to kill himself. His thinking was disorganized and he was flooded with intense anxiety over what was happening to him. An initial episode of schizophrenia can present this way, with a rapid onset of symptoms of severe psychosis and agitation, and young males appear to be more susceptible to these very severe episodes. David was 19 or 20 years old. He lived with his parents in a nearby rural county, and had been a quiet boy, without any history of acting out behaviors, prior to the onset of his symptoms. His parents were very concerned about him and wanted to see him as soon as they got to the hospital. Instead, I talked with them for a while, about what was happening to him, but did not allow them to see him, as I was afraid that it would be too dangerous. I let them know that he had a serious mental illness, and that he would likely require inpatient care for quite some time. They could not provide any information on possible precipitating events that might have contributed to the onset of his illness.

When he realized that he would not be allowed out of the seclusion room until he was able to control his behavior, he became threatening. He refused to take the medications that I prescribed for him, so I ordered that he be given IM medications until he was calmer. It took the male CNAs from both Davis units, with the assistance of other nursing staff to hold him down until the injection was given to him. I started him on high doses of Thorazine, with some Cogentin to prevent muscle side effects. I also gave him fairly high doses of Librium to try to calm him down from the severe anxiety he had. He continued to require frequent injections of the medications with the attendant necessity of staff to hold him down to administer the shots. Yet he was showing no improvement in his condition.

His psychotic symptoms were painful to watch and he remained in the seclusion room with one of the male CNAs watching him through the window all the time. We had removed the hospital bed from the room so that he would not harm himself by banging his head on the metal frame. All he had in the room at that point was a mattress on the floor. He was in a hospital gown. He would hit himself in the head at times and at other times he would pull on his hair, while shaking his head, in a vain attempt to escape the voices which were very threatening to him and continued to tell him to kill himself and others. Seeing his continuous agony as he tried to free himself from his hallucinations and paranoid fears left us feeling helpless to provide him with any relief. The other patients were also very concerned about him, as they could hear him screaming at the voices and at times making threats to kill the staff if we didn't get him out of the seclusion room.

He had arrived on the unit in the late afternoon. In spite of the medications that he had been given, he did not sleep at all that night. Many of the other patients were also unable to sleep because of the screams that came out of the seclusion room throughout the night. He finally fell asleep around 6 a.m., but even then his sleep was restless and he frequently made moaning sounds in his sleep; he also tossed and turned almost continuously. The screams had stopped however, and the unit was relatively quiet that morning.

The central issue in the morning meeting was how to deal appropriately with David and what our options were. I had already talked with the ward attending about the situation. Both of us felt that we were not going to be able to manage him on the unit because of his dangerous and out of control behaviors and his lack of response to the medications and to the containment in the seclusion room. He seemed to be the kind of patient that really required the expertise of the state hospital staff, who usually treated the severely psychotic patients who were unmanageable on the units that treated the higher functioning patients. We discussed the situation at length during the morning meeting. I outlined for the group my discussion with the attending and the option of sending him to the state hospital for acute treatment and stabilization of his psychosis. Everyone in the meeting, staff and patients, felt very concerned about him and distressed that we had not been able to help him. Some of the longer-term patients could remember other patients arriving in a severely agitated and/or psychotic state, and seeing those patients improve rapidly with the medications they received acutely. They did not want to see David sent off to the state hospital, as they felt this would be giving up on him too soon. They wanted to see him improve and be able to receive the therapeutic help that they had gotten in the culture of the unit. Most all of them were on medications and it was very anxiety provoking for them to see someone who did not respond to the medications with at least some improvement. The staff was also feeling helpless, as was I, and feeling we would be failing him if we sent him to the state hospital so quickly.

There were a few patients who acknowledged that they were very afraid of him, because of the threats he made repeatedly when he was screaming to be let out of the seclusion room. He was out of the room briefly, with both male orderlies assisting him to use the toilet, which was outside the seclusion room, but right beside it. One of the orderlies would be in the bathroom with him, while the other remained outside the door to prevent him from escaping onto the unit until he was safely back in the seclusion room. He had to be calmer to be allowed to go to the bathroom and this would occur only after he had calmed down enough to agree to just using the bathroom and then returning back to the seclusion room. All the orderlies were very good with him and they would talk to him at times when he was somewhat less agitated. But these times did not last long and were never predictable enough to let him out of the room except with very close supervision and only very briefly. The screaming and threats would usually start again as soon as he was back in the seclusion room, but he remained reasonably cooperative during the times he was out to use the bathroom. He was offered food and drink, and would sometimes eat or drink some of what was offered. The orderly sometimes stayed with him in the seclusion room while he ate, and he would appear under better control some of those times. Most of the time however, he would throw the food or drink at the wall or floor and the orderly would have to get out of the room quickly. The mess was usually cleaned up quickly, during one of the times he was in the bathroom or when he was restrained for injections.

The patients who were afraid of him were mainly afraid that he would escape out onto the unit and hurt one of them. Some of them could remember a young male sociopath who was in the seclusion room several months previously, because he would not stay out of other patients' rooms and was always stealing their things. He was a master lock pick and so he was only in a hospital gown with a mattress on the floor when he was placed in the seclusion room while we tried to decide what to do with him. He would always agree to abide by the unit rules when confronted with a recent theft, but was stealing again within the hour, when his previous stays in the seclusion room were up. With his last placement in the seclusion room, in a hospital gown and with only a mattress on the floor, he grinned as he went in and told us we would not be able to keep him there for very long. We thought he was just being defiant. But, no, he had found a way to pick the lock and was out of there in about seven hours. He was very pleased with himself. We were clearly not making any progress with him and we ended up transferring him back to his family's custody with a recommendation that they send him back to jail until his trial date on charges of felony theft and breaking and entering. The patients who could remember how this young sociopath had found a way to escape from the room, were afraid that David would also be able to escape and talked about not feeling safe with him on the unit, because he was clearly potentially dangerous if he was not continuously contained in the seclusion room. After much discussion it was decided that David should be transferred to the state hospital for the acute care he needed. I indicated that it was possible to have him transferred back to our unit once he was stable, and that he would be more likely to be able to take part in the therapeutic activities on the unit once he was more stable, and would be more likely to benefit from them at that point. The group felt better about deciding that transfer to the state hospital was the best option for him at that time, once they could see it as a part of the treatment that he needed, with him still having a chance at additional treatment on our unit when that was appropriate.

The staff felt that the state hospital was the most appropriate placement for him. We had certainly transferred other similar patients to the state hospital in Staunton, Virginia, when they had presented with severe psychosis and the potential for dangerous, out of control and violent behaviors. In fact, we had one of the other senior residents almost stabbed by a similarly psychotic patient about six months prior to David's admission. This incident had occurred on Davis II, but some of the patients on Davis III were aware of that incident, as it was discussed quite a bit on both units after it happened. That patient had come into another patient's room while one of the nurses was helping this woman cut some fabric that she wanted to use for the quilt she was making. The patient had only recently been allowed out on the unit and he had seemed to be stable on his medications. He had been in seclusion for a time due to threatening behaviors towards others, but appeared under good control at that time. He unexpectedly ran into the room, grabbed the scissors from the nurse and ran out into the hall, where he attempted to stab the resident, who was talking to one of the other nurses about another patient. The male orderly happened to be nearby and grabbed this man before he could get to the resident. The resident had been standing with his back to the patient, and was unaware of the danger until the orderly had already taken the scissors away from the patient, and had him in a tight hold with the assistance of the nurse who had been using the scissors. It was a close call and this patient was then transferred to the state hospital, because it was too dangerous to keep him on the unit any longer.

Our staff continued to feel a lot of concern for David, and we were very open to taking him back once he was stable. All of us were hopeful that he would come around and be capable of taking part in the activities and therapies we could provide when he returned. I had the first year resident set up a meeting with David's parents and we discussed the reasons that we were making the transfer to the state hospital, and our willingness to have him return to our unit once he was stable enough. They were understanding of the plan as they too had been frightened of his potential for violence. He had been a good worker on their small farm and was very strong because of all the heavy labor he had done at home. They were glad that we wanted to take him back once he was stable.

He remained at the state hospital for about four months. He had stabilized with the medication combination they had him on after six or eight weeks. He had not caused any problems in the state hospital for the two months prior to his transfer back to us. We were all looking forward to his return. And we were all very sad to see what he was like when he did return. His affect was very flat and he interacted only when approached by others. He did not initiate contact with any of the patients or the staff. He had gained about 50 pounds, which was most likely due to side effects of his medication. But, what was most sad to see for me was that his eyes were utterly empty. Since that time I have seen a large number of schizophrenic patients who get only a partial improvement with the medications. Many of them were young men, who appear to burn out emotionally with their first episode of the illness, and they remain flat and unemotional from then on. Generally they are not a risk for violent behaviors after that, and in many instances, they did not have the dangerous agitation and threats of violence that David had. But once you see the empty eyes, you can be sure that they have had severe damage from the illness that has become known as the negative symptoms of schizophrenia. David was not a problem on the unit and he would take part in a limited way in the activities on the unit. The rest of the time, he either sat and rocked in the rocking chair that was in the day room or went back to his room and laid on his bed.

David's parents were very sad to see how he had changed. He made no real progress during his second stay in the therapeutic community and after 10 or 11 weeks, his parents requested that we consider discharging him back to his home. There was a mental health center in his home county and he could be followed up on an outpatient basis there. They would also provide a case manager for him and involve him in a possible sheltered workshop if he was willing. We made no changes in the medications that he was on from the state hospital. We had him go home for a weekend pass, which went as well as could be expected. We then discharged him as the family had requested. He was agreeable to being discharged and returning home. I was left with the distinct feeling that it no longer mattered to him whether he was at home or on the unit. It was this patient, more than any other, who taught me that there are some illnesses that cannot be improved with medications and active inpatient or outpatient treatment. Patients like David appear to reach a certain level with their illness that makes them essentially unavailable emotionally to the people around them, even people that they cared about prior to their illness. They will always be very low functioning and the state hospitals could provide a very humane and safe supportive environment for these very vulnerable people.

Even now I do not believe that the deinstitutionalizing of these people has been beneficial for them. The movie *Slingblade* tells a very poignant story of someone like this, although the man in the movie was higher functioning than David was when we sent him home. But he could not deal effectively with the outside world and there are many of these patients who have essentially been abandoned by the system when the long-term institutions were closed down. People like David can make it while there are still family members who can take care of them. Without that they are very vulnerable to being homeless, with all the risks associated with that. They frequently will go without their medications under those circumstances. They may become addicted to alcohol or street drugs. They may also be assaulted or exploited by some of the more violent persons who are homeless. Many of them also commit criminal acts, frequently related to substance abuse or violence if they are more psychotic, and end up institutionalized in the criminal justice system. Those outcomes are much more damaging and dangerous for them than the state hospitals ever were.

Schizophrenia is in many ways the most severe and debilitating mental illness and it has an early age of onset for many of its victims. It was known as dementia praecox (premature dementia) when it was described in some of the early writings on psychiatric illnesses, especially the writings on psychotic illnesses. It had a poor prognosis and many of the people who suffered from this illness were committed to state hospitals and most of them remained there for the rest of their lives. Even manic-depressive disorder was considered to have a reasonably good prognosis long term, in that many of its victims were able to recover and leave the hospital, after perhaps four to five years of inpatient treatment.

In the late 1950s and early 1960s medication treatments for psychotic illnesses, including schizophrenia, became available and this is most likely what enabled the movement to deinstitutionalize long term chronically mentally ill patients back into outpatient treatment in their home communities. Sometimes they were returned to their families and sometimes they were placed in group homes or supervised apartment arrangements with case managers to closely monitor them. The medications that were initially marketed were in a class called phenothiazines and they were very effective for the treatment of what are called positive symptoms of schizophrenia, which include hallucinations, delusions, fragmented thought processes and, frequently, severe agitation. The anti-psychotic medications seemed particularly effective in decreasing severe and overwhelming anxiety which seemed to underlie the fragmentation of thinking and the distortions in their perception of reality. These medications had significant side effects, including severe weight gain and involuntary muscle movements, such as Parkinsonian muscle problems that led to a shuffling gait and limited facial expression. Later anti-psychotic medications were developed in an attempt to gain better efficacy as well as lessen the side effects. All of these medications, the older ones and the newer ones, have similar side effects and benefit for the positive symptoms of the illness. The literature from Great Britain and Europe continues to show no significant differences in the older medications as compared to the newer drugs.

These medications tend to have very limited benefit for what are called the negative symptoms of schizophrenia, which include flat affect, inappropriate affect, lack of motivation and a limited ability to engage in relationships with other people. For the most part, these are symptoms that occur in the aftermath of the initial episode of illness, and continue as a chronic aspect of the illness for the rest of their lives. There are changes in the brain, which can be demonstrated with brain scans and various types of MRIs. There is enlargement of the ventricles of the brain which is indicative of loss of brain tissue and some of these changes have been shown to pre-date the initial episode of the illness. There does appear to be an organic basis for the brain changes that accompany the symptoms of the illness. The descriptions of the emotional withdrawal from social interactions, which were attributed to the effects of being institutionalized, are in fact, an integral part of the illness, and remain evident in their behaviors, even in those patients who have not had the experience of being institutionalized for long periods of time.

This was a time of change throughout the nation and the introduction of the therapeutic community on Davis III was a part of that change. The tensions within the department were also mini-versions of the tensions being experienced and played out in the university and the broader culture of the nation. The move to deinstitutionalize the chronically mentally ill was another aspect of these developments. There were many younger people, students, interns, residents and junior staff, who were very supportive of these changes while the older staff tended to be more conservative and to see the changes as disruptive, threatening and unnecessary.

When I left for my internship in Iowa, the Department of Psychiatry was chaired be Dr. Ian Stevenson, who was doing research on reincarnation. This was not an area of research that many other people saw as a legitimate concern of psychiatry. By the time I returned to Virginia, he had stepped down as the chairman of the department, and was continuing his research with grants that supported his work. He did not do much teaching and did not attend most of the department meetings.

The new chairman was a very intelligent man who had graduated from medical school at 21 years of age, much younger than most physicians. He had advanced fairly rapidly up the academic ladder of success, and was relatively young to take over as chairman of the department. He had been at another university hospital prior to accepting the position of chairman at the University of Virginia School of Medicine Department of Psychiatry. He was ambitious and wanted to establish a strong and prestigious department. He wanted to have only American medical school graduates in his residency program. He did not like it that my residency class had several foreign born and educated physicians. It was a very diverse group, including a physician from Cuba, a physician from the Basque country of Spain and a physician from Argentina. There was also an older physician, who had been in another field of medicine for a number of years, before coming into the residency to train as a psychiatrist. The other four of us had come from an internship program and were recent medical school graduates.

The chairman had a monthly meeting for the residents. We met at his home one evening a month and we would generally talk about issues with our training and other topics related to psychiatry in general. He was generally a gracious host and, when things were going smoothly in the department, the meetings were enjoyable. He asked for honest feedback but he had difficulty hearing negative criticisms when they occurred. For instance, there was one resident in my group, who was very self-centered and also easily frustrated. He would quickly tire of the demands and challenges of whatever his new rotation was, and would then start talking about quitting the residency. He would then usually be transferred to another service that he thought would be more to his liking. Unfortunately, he usually left something of a mess behind everywhere he had been. I was pulled off my rotation on Davis II to pick up the patients he left behind on Davis III when he moved on to the consult service. I talked about the damage to patient care that sort of abrupt change could cause at the next evening with the chairman. Other residents had had similar complaints when they were abruptly pulled to another rotation and I had voiced my agreement with their concerns when they came up in previous meetings. This time I had my own personal experience with these moves, and I had

had to work very hard with two of my new patients on Davis III, in order to help them through their trust issues. I did discuss this at some length in that meeting and the chairman was noticeably colder toward me after that meeting.

By this time all of the residents were meeting one evening a month to discuss ways to try to deal with some of the problems in the residency program, problems that were impacting the morale and confidence of all of us, as we tried to become better psychiatrists in an unstable situation. Within an 18-month period we had three residents become transiently psychotic and two others who made serious suicide attempts. This took place in a resident group of 24 or 25 residents, so it was a particularly high percentage of the group.

One example of the problem occurred when there was a suicide of one of the inpatients, who had been granted a six hour pass to go home for a brief visit on a weekend day, to see if he could tolerate being with his family members for a short visit. His wife and parents were to keep someone with him throughout the visit and under no circumstances were they to leave him alone. All of this was spelled out very clearly to the patient and his family. The attending psychiatrist and the resident were both present during this discussion. The patient had been admitted following a serious suicide attempt and had been on the unit for three or four months before he was permitted this pass. In spite of all these precautions, the patient managed to separate himself from the family, gained possession of a gun, and he shot himself while he was supposedly taking his dog out for a walk before returning to the hospital.

It was always customary for there to be a meeting of the psychiatric staff and residents following a patient's suicide, to try to identify the factors that contributed to the completed suicide. Clinical staff, especially residents or nursing staff, were sometimes scapegoated in these meetings. In this patient's case the issue had come down to trying to prepare the patient for transition to outpatient status, since his inpatient insurance benefits were approaching an end in two more months, and neither he nor his family members wanted him sent to the state hospital when those benefits ran out. It was clear that the family was ambivalent about this patient's need for very close supervision and they did not comply with his psychiatrist's very clear directions not to leave him alone under any circumstances during that visit.

The resident was the one who wrote and signed the order for the pass and he became the target for the harsh criticism that the chairman and several other attendings had for the decision to give the man a brief pass to his home. The attending, who was equally responsible for the decision, had met with the patient and his family members with the resident also present, on a Friday. The pass was implemented on the following day, Saturday, for six hours during the afternoon, and the order was written on Saturday, by the resident, since the attending was out of town that day. The attending psychiatrist did accept responsibility for the decision that was made, but the resident was the one who was blamed for not withdrawing the permission for the pass, even though there were no changes in the patient's status on Saturday that would have warranted keeping him in the hospital that day.

By the time the meeting was over the resident was very paranoid and depressed. He was one of the foreign trained residents in my year, and several of us suspected that that was the reason he was treated so badly during the meeting. The meeting took place in the conference room at the mental health center, since this was the largest conference room in the psychiatric department. One of the senior residents, myself and two other residents in my year, pulled the resident, who was transiently psychotic at that point, into one of the vacant offices in the mental health center as soon as the meeting was over. He was paranoid, humiliated, depressed and enraged in the aftermath of being singled out as the one responsible for this patient's suicide, and we spent the better part of two hours talking him down from the most intense feelings he had about what had just happened. He admitted to suicidal feelings of his own during and just after the meeting. He did not want to talk to any of the attending staff, because he did not think any of them were to be trusted. We suggested one or two of the attending staff, who, we felt, could help him deal with the intense feelings he had in this situation. He still refused to consider doing that as we ended the time with him. We had been very supportive of him, as any one of us could have been caught in the same bind and he was only writing an order that had been decided on the day before, while he and his attending met with the patient and his family. I don't know if he later decided to talk with one of the attendings that we suggested. He was calmer when he left the center and was no longer suicidal. He was able to continue in the residency program and he finished in good standing.

During the late spring of my third year, 1970, there was a conference scheduled for the whole department to last two to three days, to discuss where the department stood with respect to the various treatment and educational programs. This was supposed to lead to the development of additional programs, with an eye to becoming one of the top psychiatric programs in the South, if not in the nation.

This opportunity led our resident group to meet two or three times before the department meeting was to occur. Every part of the staff, including residents and nursing staff, were to be allowed to present our assessments of the overall functioning of the department and to suggest issues to be addressed at the meeting. I agreed to present the residents' statement and I made lots of notes as the discussions unfolded around all the difficulties that each of us had faced during our time in the residency. I then summarized the issues in a 10-page paper, which I read to the resident group at our last meeting before the conference. I asked for corrections and additions, but the paper was felt to be a very accurate summation of the issues from the residents' point of view. The nurses apparently got wind of what we were doing and they came up with their own summation of issues affecting the nursing staff and their concerns about the impact of some of the dysfunction on the patients. These dysfunctional patterns were beginning to become more obvious through the feedback we were getting more directly from the patients. We had started the therapeutic community by then and the patients were empowered to speak their minds about situations on the unit that they felt needed to be handled better.

The conference started with several complimentary statements from other faculty and administrative staff and there were some self-congratulatory trends emerging in the early presentations. I then presented the concerns of the residents, to be followed by the nurse who presented the concerns of the nursing staff. The chairman was taken completely by surprise and appeared shocked and somewhat angry, though he kept that in check. We were to break up into small groups following the presentations and the focus of all the groups was on the last presentations. There were no more self-congratulations at that point and serious discussions were going on at all levels, with the younger attending staff now voicing many of their own concerns. The conference was able to address a number of the major concerns and there was no retaliation against those of us who had presented honest concerns during the presentations. The chairman was somewhat subdued in the aftermath of the meeting.

By the time of the conference, I had decided to apply to the Washington Psychoanalytic Institute for training to become a psychoanalyst. I knew that I would likely have to move to D.C. to do the training. However, it was very late in the year to apply for classes starting in the fall of 1970. I was starting to learn a lot about what is genuinely therapeutic in a treatment setting since taking over as the senior resident in the therapeutic community. I wanted to continue the work there for another year, while I prepared to start psychoanalytic training. I discussed this with two of my supervisors and they were very supportive of me staying on for a fourth year of residency and to continue to work in the therapeutic community. I then talked with the chairman about staying on for another year. He said he would consider it. Two days later he called me into his office and not only granted me a fourth year of residency, but asked me to be the chief resident as well. I agreed to do it and was able to continue learning about the therapeutic community as well as taking on some administrative responsibilities in the department, particularly in being allowed to work closely with the younger residents and medical students, which was challenging but very satisfying.

CHAPTER EIGHT

Residency: The Fourth Year

During the year I was chief resident I continued to work part-time in the therapeutic community. I had a small office on the unit and continued to see some outpatients there. I was also appointed to the faculty as an instructor in psychiatry and did some teaching as well. The psychiatrist who had been the attending on the unit had transferred to another service, working at the mental health center and I was the attending on the unit. We had a new senior resident as well as three first year residents and I was their direct supervisor as well. The nursing and treatment staff were more experienced and the unit fell into a routine pattern of meetings and activities. We continued the staff meetings, which had been the origin of the therapeutic community to start with and there was continued clinical growth for all of us with this support. I know from my own experience that there was personal growth from that experience as well. The therapeutic benefits from our work were not limited just to the patients we were treating. The residents' monthly meetings continued and there continued to be strong support for each of us from that group as well.

The chairman of the department was my direct supervisor and we were to meet weekly for an overview of the current issues with all the programs in the department. The meetings were difficult for him for reasons that were never clear to me. I was reasonably comfortable with my level of responsibilities within the department.

He was accommodating when we were working out my schedule for starting my analysis with a training analyst in Washington, D.C., which I would need to start prior to starting classes at the Washington Psychoanalytic Institute. This involved my going to D.C. for sessions in the late afternoon on Mondays and Thursdays, staying overnight in a private home on those days, then having an early morning session on Tuesdays and Fridays before returning to Charlottesville by late morning and then taking up my duties in the department for the remainder of those days. I was on backup call except for the overnights in D.C., but rarely had to come in at that point. I was accepted to the Institute to start training in the fall of 1971 and needed to have been in my personal analysis for at least 6 months prior to starting classes. On the advice from two of my supervisors, regarding which of the training analysts they would recommend for me, I was able to get an analyst that both had highly recommended, and who was a good fit for me. I started my analysis in late November of 1970 and I was able to get good coverage for my responsibilities while I was in D.C.

My meetings with the chairman were on Wednesday mornings and I was usually there by eight o'clock, which was when we were to meet. He was usually a few minutes late early on, which gave me time to get a cup of coffee from one of the units before the meeting started. As time went on he was later and later getting to the meetings and this became noticeably worse after I started my analysis. I would sit outside his office talking with his secretary until he arrived. She was very much aware of the things going on in the department and we would talk mostly about whatever the current issues were. This was one of the ways I stayed on top of what was going on in the department. By the end of the year, he was late enough that we usually met for only 10 or 15 minutes.

The only exception to that was when he came in on time for the meeting and informed me that one of the senior residents had made a serious suicide attempt the previous evening and was hospitalized on the neurology floor, under suicide precautions. He was to start treatment with one of the more senior attendings while he was hospitalized. The chairman asked me to see him and continue to monitor his status while he was in the hospital. He was clearly very worried about the resident and the impact of his attempt on his ability to return to his training within the department. I was stunned by the news as he was one of our best residents and none of us had seen any indication of depression in him. No one was aware of his suicidal impulses. I did follow up with him over the next few days and he was making good progress with his therapist. He was no longer suicidal and I indicated that I saw no reason not to have him return to his work within a week of his being discharged from the hospital.

Nathan

The resident, whom I will call Nathan, who made the serious suicide attempt, had actually graduated from UVA Medical School about two years before I did. As with all the male students at that time, he had had to serve two years in the military before going on with his training. The nation was in the initial stages of building up the troops in Vietnam when he graduated in 1964. This was during President Lyndon Johnson's administration and a lot of young men were being drafted into the military if they were not in college. This was before the draft lottery was instituted a few years later. For the average American man, if you had not been drafted by the age of 26, you were essentially exempt from the draft at that point. However, if you went to medical school and graduated, you were eligible for the draft up to the age of 40. All of my classmates, except for myself and the other two women, had to make arrangements for additional training in some way that would fit with the time they would have to serve in the military.

Nathan had been with the Army Air Corps, and was stationed stateside in North Carolina. He had talked about his time in the service with me and seemed to be satisfied with the situation he had been in. He was an excellent resident when he came back as a first year resident. He was thoughtful and did good work with his patients; he was also active in the residents' meetings. He even organized a bowling team for

165

interested residents. I joined the team and we were one of the league teams in duckpin bowling for my third year of residency. It was a lot of fun. I had never bowled and was terrible at the beginning. By the end of the year I was doing much better and won the "most improved bowler" designation for the league that year. Most of us on the team were single and I do not think Nathan was in a relationship during that year.

He seemed to have everything together, so I was really stunned to hear of his suicide attempt. I went by to talk to him in the afternoon after I heard about it. He told me that he had been depressed for some time and had been suicidal much of that time. When I let him know that he did not appear depressed during the time he was on the units, he admitted that he did everything he could to hide the depression when he was with others. I said that must have left him exhausted and drained at the end of the day, and he was surprised that I knew that. Then I disclosed to him that I had also had severe depressive episodes since the age of 17 and that I always hid mine from others as well. I was very familiar with the emotional cost of that situation. Then he told me in detail about his attempt.

His sister and brother-in-law had visited with him for a few days and he was feeling more and more drained by the need to keep his depression hidden from them. When they left he went immediately to get his gun with every intention of shooting himself in the heart. His brother-in-law unexpectedly came back in to get something that he had forgotten, and found Nathan with the gun pointing at his heart. Nathan pulled the trigger, but he had not yet taken off the safety. His brother-in-law tackled him as he was struggling to get the safety off, and got the gun away from him. He then called for help and notified the attending psychiatrist of the situation.

The chairman was notified and he, the attending on call and the supervising psychiatrist on the unit Nathan was currently working on came to his home and stayed with him until they could make arrangements for Nathan to be admitted to the hospital on the neurology service under close supervision. Nathan described how he was pretending to go along with the arrangements while at the same time trying to think of anything else in his home that he could kill himself with before the three of them could stop him. He had decided to try to stab himself with a kitchen knife, but could not move away from them quickly enough to get the knife and stab himself before they would stop him. They got the arrangements made within 45 minutes and he ran out of time to try anything else at his home. He admitted to still having some thoughts about how to kill himself while on the unit, but the impulses were not as intense by then. He had met with the psychiatrist who would be his therapist and had felt really understood while talking with him. He felt, for the first time, that he might be able to get through his depression, but was almost afraid to let himself have hope.

I shared with him my own long-term depression and chronic suicidal ideation. My plan was to inject myself with a lethal dose of morphine or one of the other opiates and I'd thought about that off and on for about seven or eight years. Like Nathan, I planned to do something that would be quickly lethal, with no chance of failing. I told him how upset I was during the lecture on narcotic antagonists, when I learned that

I could be saved if someone found me in time. I told him that I left the lecture thinking that I needed to develop a better plan. We both had a laugh at that and he told me that he had been very angry with himself over failing to succeed with shooting himself; particularly during the time the senior psychiatrists were making the arrangements for his hospitalization. I could completely sympathize with him on that. We then got into one of those black comedy moments when we were both trying to out do the other in thinking through and proposing more and more extreme ways to do ourselves in so that no one could stop us. By that time we were both laughing so hard that we were gasping for breath and our stomach muscles were hurting. It was truly hysterical and a great relief at the same time.

After we calmed down, he talked for a few minutes about his anxiety about being in therapy, an anxiety that I had strongly feared as well, and his surprise at the relief he had felt after talking with his therapist. By then I had been in my own analysis for about four months, and was already experiencing a lot relief in beginning to get at the origins of my own depression. I shared with him the benefits that I had gotten from the sensitivity group I had been in during my third year of residency, and the way that facilitated my being able to get into my own treatment with the analysis during my fourth year of residency. I told him that I had even picked out the hospital I would go to if I got severely depressed and suicidal during the analysis. I wanted to give it every chance of success and even at that early point, I did not think I was going to have to use the hospital and I told Nathan that.

I left shortly after that, feeling very good about his situation and also my own. We did not talk about that time again during the remainder of the year that I was in the residency. I think that open discussion, about our depressions and the intense suicidal impulses, was helpful for both of us. He completed his residency and returned to his hometown in southern Virginia to set up practice. I heard about him occasionally from others who had been in medical school or residency with us. He had married and had a family. He also had a busy and successful practice. The last I heard, he had retired and was enjoying his retirement.

For me, it was a relief to be able to talk to a colleague about my own struggles with depression and suicide. It confirmed, in a different way, that I made the right choice to enter my own analysis. I had also been accepted to the psychoanalytic institute and so was officially doing the analysis as a requirement for that training. However, I was very clear, and I was able to let my analyst know after my time with Nathan, that my personal treatment was why I was there, and the training was always going to be secondary to the analysis. My analyst had no difficulty accepting that. He indicated that my attitude made it more likely that I would get the best result from my treatment and that I also would likely gain more from the training, since I was so open to my own need for the treatment. Two years later he was able to send a report to the institute that I had completed the necessary work in my analysis, meeting all the criteria necessary for that part of my training. It was another two and a half years before I actually completed the analysis, and I did get an exceptionally good result from that treatment.

The last time I had any significant mood symptoms was just prior to my starting the analysis. Through this process, I learned to accept my important losses and learned to grieve those losses, which was the most critically important benefit from the treatment. I have no doubt that the analysis saved my life and I have remained very grateful for that healing relationship, which resolved the issues that had made me suicidal so many times during my late teens and most of my twenties. It has also left me very respectful of the patients I treat, because I understand how difficult it is to trust your most intimate issues and concerns with someone else, even someone whose responsibility it is to help you gain mastery over those issues.

The chairman and I remained on cordial but distant terms during my last year of residency; he wished me well in my analytic training when I left at the end of the year. I moved to Falls Church, Virginia to work at the Northern Virginia Mental Health Institute, start a practice and begin my psychoanalytic training.

Occasionally I received news from the department after I moved and eventually learned that the chairman resigned from the department after several more years. He was never able to build the kind of department that he had wanted to. He also did not appear to be comfortable with the newer trends in the department, that allowed for more active participation and planning by the patients in the therapeutic community, as well as with the students, residents and the younger faculty members. I ran into him several years later at one of the American Psychiatric Association meetings. We had a discussion about what we had been doing since we last met at the end of my residency. I was well into my psychoanalytic training at that time and I was enjoying it very much. He was now in charge of the consult-liaison service in one of the teaching hospitals in the Midwest and he seemed to be more comfortable in that situation. He was more subdued than he had been during the time he was chairman. We parted on a good note and I felt some closure with that relationship.

CHAPTER NINE

State Hospital Therapeutic Community

After completing my fourth year of residency, I moved to Falls Church, Virginia to begin work at the Northern Virginia Mental Health Institute in Fairfax, Virginia. This hospital had opened within the previous two years as an acute care hospital. The length of stay on average was between four and six months. If someone was not ready to leave the hospital by the time their insurance for mental health treatment was up or at around six months, they would then be transferred to the long-term state hospital, Western State Hospital in Staunton, Virginia. There were six units in the hospital in Fairfax, and they had already adopted the therapeutic community model for most of the units. With my experience running the therapeutic community on Davis III for sixteen months, I was able to transition to the new hospital without any difficulty.

During the six months I worked at the Northern Virginia Mental Health Institute, I was able to continue working with a therapeutic community, in much the same way I had done with the similar unit on Davis III. We had the morning meetings of staff and patients to discuss current issues and to decide changes in patients' status on the unit, including home passes. The staff worked well together and the patient group was working hard on their own issues in a context of a general respect for their needs and their healing process. I will give one example of the process, which was very characteristic of how this unit functioned.

Gina

Shortly after I arrived on the unit, we admitted a patient, whom I will call Gina, who was acutely ill with her initial episode of schizophrenia. She was acutely agitated and psychotic at first, and was too ill to take part in the morning meetings. She responded fairly rapidly to the Stelazine that I had started her on, and her hallucinations and delusions cleared fairly quickly. She was then much calmer, but was showing a lot of the negative symptoms of schizophrenia. Her affect was very flat and she needed a lot of encouragement to take part in the activities on the unit. She had no initiative and would have stayed in bed in her room if staff and other patients had not kept after her to take part in the activities. She was a young woman, in her very early thirties, and she was married to a man who genuinely cared for her. She seemed almost indifferent to him when he visited her on the unit, and she seemed to have difficulty talking to him in any kind of spontaneous way. He was working for a government subcontractor and he had good federal insurance coverage for her. She had four months of inpatient coverage, but would have to go to the state hospital in Staunton, if she did not recover enough to return home. He reported that she was nothing like she had been prior to the onset of her illness. She had been rather quiet but appeared to get along well with friends and family. He reported that the marriage had been good before her illness.

After about three weeks, she began to attend the morning meetings with the rest of the patients and the staff. She did not take part in the discussions, and usually sat huddled in the corner of one of the couches in the day room, which is where the meetings were held. She did interact somewhat with her roommate and with a few of the other patients outside of the meetings, but for the most part she stayed to herself unless approached by someone else. The social worker on the unit met with her and her husband several times, but she was always uncomfortable during these meetings. They did not have children and Gina said that she could not have cared for children with her illness. Her husband had been very hopeful that she would return to her previous self, especially when the hallucinations and delusions cleared so rapidly with the medication. But as time went on, and she did not make any additional improvements, he became more concerned about whether she would be able to leave the hospital when her insurance benefits ran out. When he raised these concerns with her, she indicated that she wanted to go to the state hospital in Staunton, because she did not feel she could keep up with her responsibilities at home that she once did without difficulty. When the other patients would try to encourage her to try to work toward going home, she would become anxious and withdraw from them as soon as she could.

As she was approaching her last three weeks of insurance coverage, the other patients were talking to her a lot about how she needed to try to return home. By this time her husband was feeling very disheartened by her lack of progress and her emotional distance from him, and he was not visiting her as often as he did at first. Patients and staff were trying to motivate her to work harder toward returning home to her husband. She was becoming more and more miserable as she felt everyone on the unit was against her. Increasing the dosage of her Stelazine did nothing to change the negative symptoms. She was getting significant weight gain from the medication and by the end of her hospitalization, she had gained almost 50 pounds, all of which appeared to be secondary to side effects from the medication.

With about 10 days left for her hospitalization, she came into the morning meeting, looking very anxious and miserable. She took her usual place on the couch, and she was clearly trying to hide behind the patient who was sitting next to her on the couch. I was sitting part way down the circle from her and I could not see her without leaning forward in my seat. Gina's situation was the main topic of concern that day, with almost everyone talking about how important it was for her to be able to return home when she was discharged. She made no response to any of the comments by the other patients or the staff. As I listened to the discussion I suddenly remembered Frannie, and her need for the longer-term hospitalization. And I realized that Gina was not going to be able to return home. Her affect was still very flat, she was emotionally distant and she was easily overwhelmed, by even minor stressors. Her eyes were empty for the most part and she couldn't really change what had happened to her when she became psychotic.

So I started to tell the group about my session with Frannie, describing in detail how she had been bedfast and unresponsive for ten months, before she began to recover. I described how difficult it was for her to deal with everyday life when she left the protection of the state hospital, even with the support of her aunt and uncle. She had spent several years in the state hospital before she reached a point where she was ready to venture into the regular world again. I described how she had been aware of the people around her during the time she was immobilized, but could not make the effort to communicate with them. Initially she had been afraid of everything, but after a while she was less afraid of her caregivers on the staff because they were kind to her. She felt safe after a time and that was when she began to respond and interact with others again. I came to the point in the story when I asked her, "Why do you think you did that for so long?" I talked about how she had thought for several minutes before replying. Then she said, "I'm not sure. I just needed that time."

As I said those last words, the male patient, who was sitting beside me, elbowed me gently in the arm, and he said, "Look at Gina." I leaned forward to see her and she was sitting on the edge of the couch, looking at me intently, and she was smiling as she looked me in the eye. She was nodding her head, and she said, "That's it. That's what I need." It was the most animated she had been since her admission, and she no longer had to hide from me or the other group members. The rest of the group began to talk in supportive ways about her need to go to the longer-term state hospital and they could now understand why that was necessary for her. The whole focus of the community changed and for the remainder of the time on the unit, her decision was accepted and respected. She was able to interact a bit more with staff and patients. She appeared to be more at ease on the unit. The social worker met with Gina and her husband shortly before she was to leave for the hospital in Staunton. He seemed sad but resigned to seeing her go to the longer-term hospital.

On the day that she left, the other patients came to her room, one or two at a time, and they wished her well. She seemed to derive some benefit from the support she was receiving. She received hugs from most of the patients as she was leaving. She had a small smile on her face as she left the unit. The therapeutic community had been able to focus on what she wanted and, which, by then, I felt was what she really needed, and accept and respect her choice, given the mental devastation she had suffered from her illness. The patients and staff could genuinely wish her well in the new treatment environment she was entering and feel hopeful for her in the long run. There was closure without blame or a sense of failure, and this was a truly healing experience for all of us in the community.

Katherine

While most of the patients we treated were able to respond to the treatment and return to their previous lives, there were still some issues that required unusual interventions. Because we were located in northern Virginia, we frequently treated patients who were government employees and some of them were in jobs that required high-level security clearances. When one of these patients was hospitalized we would get two agents that we informally thought of as "suits" or "spooks" and we knew we had to give them an accurate account of the patient's ability to protect the highly classified information they were privy too and also whether they would be able to return to the agency they worked for once they were discharged. One of these patients, a woman in her 50s whom I will call Katherine, was a government employee who had a very high security clearance and as was usual in such situations, we had a visit from two men from one of the government agencies to make sure she was not disclosing any government secrets. Her job was clearly on the line but it was also clear that she was a valued employee with an uncommon skill set. She worked for one of the intelligence agencies and spent all of her time on the job in a locked room by herself, receiving and decoding messages for the agency. It was clearly a question of whether her illness rendered her unable to protect the classified information that she handled on a daily basis. Katherine was one of five to seven individuals with this high level of security clearance that I have personally treated and not one of them has disclosed any of this classified information, not even the four or five that were severely psychotic. The ability to maintain these secrets had always remained intact even with the psychosis.

She had been admitted acutely with the recent onset of a psychotic illness and she was having hallucinations and delusions. She had no prior history of serious mental illness, but did have a history of episodic depression, which she had handled without seeking treatment. She was hearing voices and also had the delusion that aliens were inserting thoughts in her brain through electrical transmissions from Mars. Katherine had been very agitated and paranoid at the time of her admission and had the racing thoughts characteristic of a manic episode. She was started on one of the anti-psychotic medications (lithium was not yet available in the states) and she had a good response to the medication, with fairly rapid clearing of the agitation and hallucinations, though she continued to show manic symptoms of racing thoughts, decreased sleep and a high energy and activity level. She was able to take part in individual therapy sessions as well as the other activities on the unit. She talked about some recent stressors within her family that she was very upset about. This had to do with problems with two of her adult children who were going through severe problems in their marriages and it looked as if both marriages were going to end in divorce. The patient had divorced their father when they were relatively young and she had continued to raise them as a single mother into adulthood. There was at least one grandchild that would be affected with one of the divorces and she was very distressed about this. She also felt somehow responsible for her children's marital difficulties since she had been unable to salvage her own marriage and her ex-husband had not maintained a reliable relationship with their children after her divorce. The social worker met with her and her children on several occasions during her hospitalization, helping her to begin to process these issues. Gradually, she began to improve and was approaching discharge after two months of treatment. She was very anxious to return to her job as soon as she could. She was very good at it and tolerated being in the room by herself and actually liked that part of the job. She enjoyed the work and knew she was doing important work. She derived a lot of personal satisfaction from her work.

We had been visited by the two agents early in her hospitalization and at that time I had been able to tell them that she was not a security risk as a result of her illness since her persecutors were on Mars and there had been no mention of her work at all during the early stages of her illness. They returned shortly before her discharge and I was able to tell them that she was making a good recovery from a manic episode and that she would need to continue on the medication to prevent a relapse. I discussed with them in a general way the family problems that had precipitated her breakdown. All of her psychotic symptoms had cleared by then. I reassured them that she did not discuss her job beyond a very basic description of her responsibilities and there were no disclosures of any of the classified information she knew at any time during her treatment, even the times she was psychotic. I recommended that she return to her work within a week of being discharged from the hospital. They accepted my recommendation and indicated her clearance still remained in place. She did return to work without any problems and continued to see an outpatient psychiatrist for her medication follow-up.

Eddie

The next young man, whom I will call Eddie, was another one of my patients at the Northern Virginia Mental Health Institute. At just 19 or 20 years old, he was another young man who had one of those devastating initial episodes of schizophrenia. Unlike David, his illness came on somewhat more gradually and he did not experience much in the way of hallucinations. They cleared quickly once he was started on one of the anti-psychotic medications. He was from a rural area northwest of the D.C. suburbs, and had been somewhat low functioning prior to the onset of his illness. He had dropped out of eighth grade as soon as he turned 16. His family had a small farm where they raised a large garden, a small number of cattle and a flock of chickens. They had a small allotment for raising tobacco on part of the land and this was their primary cash crop. He helped out with the work on the farm and had been reliable with his chores until shortly before the onset of his illness. He began to complain initially that something was wrong with his head, but could not tell his family exactly what was wrong. Within a few days he was beginning to show confusion at times, and became very forgetful. He was no longer doing his chores and he mostly wandered around the house and yard as if he was looking for something. Then he began to talk to people who weren't there, sometimes carrying on lengthy and/or loud conversations.

He complained of hearing voices that were saying bad things about him and he began to ask his family to make the voices stop being mean to him. By then his family was very concerned about him and they took him to their local ER. He was committed to the hospital for treatment of his mental illness.

Within a few days of starting medication for his psychosis, he was no longer having auditory hallucinations. By then he was showing the classic negative symptoms of schizophrenia with flat affect, poor social interactions and lack of interest in unit activities. He had to be prompted to attend the group meetings and most of the time he would get up and wander off part way through the meeting. He continued to have a single delusion that remained fixed for the remainder of the time that he was on the unit. He was convinced that someone had taken his real head and replaced it with a new head, which was strange and didn't work right. He began to wander the unit, including entering other patients' rooms, searching for his real head. The other patients got somewhat angry with him at first, because he was invading their space, which was against unit rules. His behavior was discussed during the morning meeting and he insisted that the only reason he was in their rooms was so he could find his real head and get it put back on. He continued his wandering behaviors without any change and by then the other patients knew that he was severely ill. Many of them would take him by the hand and quietly ask him to go back to the day room with them, as he was not supposed to be there. He would allow himself to be led back to the day room without a fuss, but was usually wandering again within a few minutes. The nursing staff would also stop him in the hallway when he was on one of his searches and they would bring him back to the dayroom, sometimes spending a little time with him, trying to get him distracted and into some other activity. He remained hospitalized with us for about six weeks. He remained free of hallucinations after the first few days, but the other symptoms of his disease remained unchanged throughout the remainder of his hospitalization. After four or five weeks, I had the social worker bring his parents in for a planning meeting and we talked with him and his parents about making arrangements for him to be transferred to the state hospital in Staunton for long term care for his schizophrenia. They were initially against sending him to the long-term hospital, but after spending some time with him on the unit and seeing his constant wandering which was secondary to his delusion that someone had taken his real head, they could better understand why we made that recommendation. He had apparently had a great uncle who had been placed at Staunton many years before and he had remained there until his death. By then the family knew that Eddie had the same illness and that he was unlikely to be able to leave the long-term hospital. I indicated that if new medications became available that would improve the delusional thinking, that he might then be able to return home. They consented to the transfer to Western State and he was transferred at the end of six weeks on the unit as chronically mentally ill with schizophrenia.

While there have been numerous new medications developed for the treatment of schizophrenia, none of them have been that effective for the negative symptoms of the disease. And they are still not always effective for all the positive symptoms either. I have seen a number of patients who continue to have chronic hallucinations and/or delusions in spite of multiple trials of medication, without success. This remains tragically the most serious and debilitating of the chronic mental illnesses. I have seen a number of patients who continue to have significant psychiatric symptoms, especially negative symptoms, who have returned home once they are stable on their medications. Family members, usually the parents, will ask for additional medication trials for their affected adult child, as they are consistently worried about the flat affect and the lack of motivation. The patients no longer seem emotionally available to others and no longer have any motivation or interest in things that they used to enjoy. In most instances, these additional medication trials do not produce any improvement in the patient. I do recommend to the family that looking for further information about the illness may be helpful, and I also acknowledge their sadness. Grief is a normal reaction to the loss of the person that they knew and loved prior to the devastating illness that so radically changed their loved one into someone they no longer feel like they know.

Unfortunately, I have seen similar issues in families when one member has suffered a severe head injury or concussion, with significant personality changes after they have recovered from the acute effects of the head injury. Significant brain damage can produce these changes, whether they occur with a severe schizophrenic episode or a physical brain injury.

The patient continues to live and interact with the family, but they will never be the same person again. This will always be a loss for the other family members who knew them before the illness or injury changed things irrevocably. Grieving that loss is a necessary part of the family's adaptation to the changed circumstances of the patient's life with the illness.

One of the senior residents that I had worked with at the mental health center had established a full time practice in Falls Church. He let me sublet his space one evening a week and on Saturdays for six or seven hours, which were times that he was not in the office. I began to develop a part-time practice, which filled up the time I had available very quickly. I was continuing to see my analyst four times a week, on the same schedule that I'd had when commuting from Charlottesville. I was to start classes at the Institute in September and the classes were on Tuesday evenings and Saturday mornings. I had to rearrange my Saturday patients to accommodate the class times on Saturday and I quickly realized that I was not going to be able to continue at the hospital on a full time basis due to the time constraints for the part-time practice and the requirements for the psychoanalytic training.

The training required that I be in my analysis, attend the classes and, shortly after starting classes, I would need to start a patient in analysis under supervision which would require meeting with my supervisor once weekly and the patient at least four times a week. While I was enjoying the work at the hospital, I was not willing to work a 60 to 70 hour work week, which was going to be required if I continued at the hospital. I put in a 60-day notice at the hospital at the end of October, to be effective on December 31, 1971. I found office space in Arlington, Virginia, which was close to the Key Bridge between Arlington and Georgetown in D.C. This gave me quick access to the Psychoanalytic Institute on MacArthur Boulevard and also quick access to downtown D.C. and DuPont Circle where my analyst had his office. When my lease on the apartment in Falls Church was up, I moved into Arlington, close to the airport, and everything was more convenient once I made that last move.

I remained in Arlington for three years and then moved into D.C., as I was able to rent an office at 3000 Connecticut Avenue, where there were a lot of other psychiatrists and psychoanalysts in practice. I bought a one-bedroom apartment in the building next door, 3100 Connecticut Avenue, and I could easily walk to the office for work. I was able to rent a parking space in the below ground parking garage of the apartment building across the street, so the car was available when I needed to go to places that were not convenient for public transportation. I could ride the bus south from my apartment building to DuPont Circle, and the group that I met with for lunch on Fridays was easily available going north on Connecticut Avenue. These moves made my schedule easier to work with and I developed a workable routine for my practice and for the analytic training. Eventually I moved out to Bethesda and moved my office to Chevy Chase. This was later, when the first four years of training at the psychoanalytic institute were completed and I had fewer supervision hours to attend. My practice consisted of psychoanalysis with about half my practice hours and intensive (one to three times a week), psychoanalytically oriented psychotherapy with the rest of the time. I still attended classes on Saturdays, but not on Tuesday evenings. This enabled me to spend more time with friends and to be involved in activities with the Washington Psychiatric Society, including being on the executive committee for two years. I was interested in getting psychiatric treatment covered by insurance, on the same basis as physical illnesses. This equal coverage has been called getting mental health parity. By the end of my two years on the committee, it was clear mental health parity was not going to happen anytime soon, and I withdrew from the political arena to focus more on personal issues.

Eventually it became clear that maintaining a psychoanalytic practice in D.C. was going to be very difficult and time consuming. The insurance companies were cutting back on coverage for mental health treatments, particularly psychoanalytic treatment, and they were also beginning to require treatment summaries on patients in order to continue to authorize additional treatment. On average, the summaries had to be done every two months. Psychoanalysis quickly became available only to those individuals who could pay out of pocket for the treatment. Even doing psychoanalytically oriented psychotherapy was more difficult, as pre-authorization for the additional treatment was usually necessary after every 10 to 12 visits. After completing my psychoanalytic training in February 1983, I decided to move to the Tri-Cities area in northeast Tennessee and southwest Virginia. By then I had adopted two sons as a single parent. I had family in the area that could provide support and it was a good area in which to start a general psychiatric practice. For the past 30 years I have maintained a small private practice and for most of that time; I have also done contract work for several different mental health organizations. At least 30% of my practice has always been with children and adolescents, with the balance including adults and some geriatric patients.

As of September 2014, I am no longer doing the contract work, but I do continue a small private practice one afternoon a week. This has opened up the time I needed to write this book and others to come.

CHAPTER TEN

Final Thoughts

A therapeutic community setting is in stark contrast to what is currently practiced in medicine, particularly involving the mentally ill. The organization of medical care in the old wards and in the newer therapeutic communities in some psychiatric hospitals was already beginning to change when I was in medical school and residency. Medicare and Medicaid came into being in 1965 as part of the War on Poverty. For a short period of time there was a lot of financial support for hospitals and physicians but this did not last. Soon pressures from the insurance companies came into play as those companies began to look to making a profit from their part in the health care industry, partly by reducing their costs for the delivery of payments for medical care. Large health care companies and facilities began to appear in place of local hospitals to take advantage of the benefits the insurance companies, Medicare and Medicaid provided for the care they could deliver. Longer-term hospitalizations for treatment began to be discouraged for physical medicine and the beginnings of pre-authorizations for psychiatric treatments followed shortly. With many services being insured now the states were interested in transferring the costs of care for the chronically mentally ill as well as the mentally retarded away from long-term state run facilities to these individuals, many of whom were indigent and who could be covered under the Medicare and Medicaid programs. They had been able to do this with the tuberculosis sanitariums when outpatient treatment for TB became possible with the effective medications that were then available.

As human beings, we have lived in communities throughout history and in smaller versions of communities in nomadic bands and tribes in prehistory. We are a social species, as are all the primates, and having a reliable community for individual and family support is something that has been essential to our well being for thousands of years. One of the ways of thinking about the care of patients in the hospital setting is to think of the wards as small specialized communities within the larger specialized community of the hospital. One of the important aspects of community is the presence of individuals that have been living and working in the community over a long period of years and who have knowledge of what works and doesn't work for the more permanent members of that community. A brilliant account of the functioning of such an urban specialized community is contained in the first three chapters of Jane Jacobs' book *The Life and Death of Great American Cities*. It is about the use of sidewalks in Greenwich Village in New York, as the transitional place in the community between the individual homes of the families who lived there and the businesses, restaurants and schools in the neighborhood, where many of them worked. She distinguished between the longer-term residents, those who worked there and the customers and visitors who were there for specific services.

A hospital unit can be thought of as a specialized community whose purpose is to provide a supportive and healing environment for people who require inpatient treatment. The long-term residents of the unit would be the nursing staff, who spend the most time on the unit and who are familiar with one another from working side by side with each other on a day-to-day basis. Doctors are there also long term, though they do not spend the same amount of time there as the nurses do. The unit interfaces with other individuals who provide additional services throughout the hospital, such as food services, laboratory services, janitorial services and so on. These individuals are generally well known to the unit staff. In the larger specialized community of a teaching hospital, there will be medical and nursing students who may spend anywhere from one to four months on the unit, assisting with the care of the patients as they learn in a hands-on way to become nurses and physicians. The patients are the individuals who are there because they need the specialized services that the hospital provides. This book has been about the learning process of a student doctor as well as the experiences that specific patients had in the hospital community during the course of their illnesses.

Intact communities depend on the presence of a stable group of individuals who maintain the structure of the community in a way that allows it to endure over time and provide for the ongoing needs of those who reside there at any given time. While the therapeutic communities I worked in for almost two years were intentionally created as communities, the other units I was on during my training years were also specialized communities without being so labeled. The backbone that the nursing staff provided on the open wards in the Iowa hospital functioned as an essential structure for the physicians, the students and the patients that were there for a more limited time. Similar situations were present on units that were set up with private, two and four bed rooms for the patients. The nurses on those units, as on all nursing units at that time, got a report at the beginning of their shift on every patient on the unit with special attention given to patients who might get into trouble during that shift. The report was done in a conference room on the unit, which provided privacy for that meeting to protect the privacy of that information.

The chart room for the doctors served a similar purpose for the physicians and students. We would frequently talk about the patients we were treating currently and could often get feedback from other doctors about what had worked for similar patients in their experience. There was an informal, spontaneous camaraderie in these exchanges that enhanced our knowledge as individual physicians as well as served as what we called "curb side consults" that were very helpful for overall patient care for many of our patients. These times could also be very supportive when we were dealing with patients who were at risk of a bad outcome or who would likely die in the hospital. These informal discussions were also done in the cafeteria, especially at midnight supper for the on call staff. All of these times helped us to get through the hard times and to gain real life experience of illnesses and problems through second hand information on patients who were not under our care. The morning rounds that were done with the students and the attending physician on the open ward or in the hallway outside patient rooms on more enclosed units were excellent learning experiences. Seeing the patients at the bedside for some of these discussions and demonstrations of physical findings was an invaluable learning experience on a daily basis. Collaborative care for our patients was readily available through these means in a way that worked very well for the patients we were responsible for. I do not believe it violated the patient's right to confidentiality as it took place in the context of an intact community that was providing specialized care and treatment in the best way possible.

I strongly believe that we have lost a lot of genuinely patient-centered care in the mistaken attempt to provide absolute confidentiality of a patient's healthcare information to the detriment of the specialized community of providers; nurses, doctors, nurse practioners, physician's assistants and students. The fragmentation of patient care, the efforts to find our way back to something resembling the old collaborative care and the relative isolation of both patient and practitioner in the treatment process are a result of the dismantling and loss of the old communities for learning and healing that shaped and supported my development as a physician and a psychiatrist. This book is presenting a history of what has worked in the past, what we have lost over the intervening years and what we may need to reconsider in the future, given the limits on resources that we will be facing within the next few decades.

Linda R. Thompson

Dr. Linda R. Thompson has been a practicing physician in the area of psychiatry since 1966, when she graduated from the University of Virginia School of Medicine. A true pioneer at the time, she was one of only three women in her med school class. She went on to complete a rotating internship at the State University of Iowa Hospital in 1967, and she returned to the University of Virginia Hospital for her residency in psychiatry from 1967-1971.

She graduated in 1983 from an extensive ten-year psychoanalytic training program at the Washington Psychoanalytic Institute, while also running an active private practice in the Washington DC area. Returning to her native East Tennessee, she maintained a general psychiatric practice serving Northeast Tennessee and Southwest Virginia from 1984 through 2014. Today, she continues to maintain a part-time general psychiatric and psychotherapy practice and devotes much of her time to writing. *Old School Medicine* is her third book.

For more information, visit Dr. Linda Thompson online:

www.tobaslegacy.com

www.ingramcontent.com/pod-product-compliance
Lightning Source LLC
Chambersburg PA
CBHW031432270326
41930CB00007B/668